PATIENT INTERVIEWING

THE HUMAN DIMENSION

PATIENT INTERVIEWING

THE HUMAN DIMENSION

David E. Reiser, M.D.
Chief, Mental Hygiene Clinic, Veteran's Administration Medical Center
San Francisco, California
Former Director, Introduction to Clinical Medicine Interviewing Course
University of Colorado Health Sciences Center
Denver, Colorado

Andrea Klein Schroder, M.S.W.
Instructor, Department of Psychiatry
Former Director, Introduction to Clinical Medicine Interviewing Course
University of Colorado Health Sciences Center
Denver, Colorado

With Contributions by

Allan R. Liebgott, M.D.
Director of Adult Medicine
Westside Neighborhood Health Program
Denver Department of Health and Hospital
Assistant Professor, Division of General Internal Medicine
Department of Medicine
University of Colorado Health Sciences Center
Denver, Colorado

Carl L. Shmock, M.D.
Associate Professor, Department of Medicine
Division of Internal Medicine
Former Director, Introduction to Clinical Medicine Interviewing Course
University of Colorado Health Sciences Center
Denver, Colorado

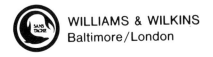
WILLIAMS & WILKINS
Baltimore/London

Reprinted 1981, 1982, 1984

Library of Congress Cataloging in Publication Data

Reiser, David E
    Patient interviewing.

    Includes index.
    1. Medical history taking. I. Schroder, Andrea Klein, joint author. II. Title.
[DNLM: 1. Interview, Psychological. 2. Medical history taking. 3. Physician-patient
relations. WB290 R375p]
RC65.R44   616.07′51   80-10567
ISBN 0-633-07226-9

Composed and printed at the
Waverly Press, Inc.
Mt. Royal and Guilford Aves.
Baltimore, Md. 21202, U.S.A.

THIS BOOK IS DEDICATED TO THE MEMORIES OF

Lorin L. Stephens, M.D. (1925–1974)

John L. Klein, M.D. (1912–1979)

FOREWORD

I am honored to have been asked to introduce the reader to this book. It is a remarkable accomplishment not simply because the authors have successfully achieved their goal of writing a text about patient interviewing. That in itself is not so unusual. A number of excellent contributions about the interviewing process have already been written, and there will be many more in the future. But there is another part to the title: "The Human Dimension." It is the attainment of that goal that makes this book so unique.

The book is divided into three parts. In Part I David Reiser sets the stage—what it is like to be a doctor, what it is like to be a patient. And he does this with great literary artistry and emotional power. Chapter 1 is a short story about a 1st year medical student and a dying patient. It is written in a fictional style, but it has the convincing ring of authenticity. In Chapters 2, 3, and 4 the reader comes to understand with even greater authenticity what it is like to be a medical student, and what it is like to be a patient. Medical training is conceptualized as a developmental stage, but so also is medical illness, for in Chapter 3 Doctor Reiser discusses his own personal experience with a serious and potentially fatal illness. This courageous chapter in and of itself elevates the book to a new "human dimension" among medical textbooks.

In Part II Dr. Reiser is joined by Andrea Klein Schroder, and together they present the interview process in a lucid and richly readable manner. Patients and interviewers come alive before our eyes, and the complex concepts of interviewing technique, process themes, and transference-countertransference patterns are once again presented in a "human dimension" that will be illuminating both to beginning interviewers and to seasoned clinicians.

In Part III Dr. Reiser is joined by Carl Shmock and Allan Liebgott. They proceed to delineate the practical issues of medical interviewing—what to look for in the medical history, how to obtain the information, how to organize the data, and then how to record it in a coherent and meaningful way. They do so in an immensely practical, common-sense manner that at the same time never loses sight of the human dignity and unique individuality of each and every patient.

The authors state in their Preface that contemporary medicine with all of its great technological advances too often seems to be preoccupied with the weakened human condition at the expense of the regenerative human spirit. This book redresses that imbalance. Anyone who has an interest in patient care, and especially anyone who deals on a firsthand basis with the medically ill, will find much here of great practical value. But beyond that, the reader will find an attitude throughout that is uplifting, perhaps even ennobling. I for one found myself deeply moved by this book.

Richard C. Simons, M.D.
Professor of Psychiatry
University of Colorado
Health Sciences Center

PREFACE

This book is an outgrowth of our experience in the Introduction to Interviewing course that we have taught at the University of Colorado Health Sciences Center. The course is part of an integrated 2-year Introduction to Clinical Medicine (ICM) sequence taught to medical students during their freshman and sophomore years.

Through a coordinated series of courses, the ICM sequence attempts to introduce beginning students to important clinical attitudes and skills that are essential to the effective functioning of a physician. The sequence begins with a broad introduction into the health care system: the social, political, and economic dimensions of the profession. Interviewing and clinical problem-solving are also begun during the 1st year. During the 2nd year students take courses in physical examination and additional clinical problem solving and finally culminate their experience with a preclerkship during the Spring quarter of their sophomore year. The goal of the preclerkship is the integration of these different clinical skills, including the interview, medical history, physical examination, write up, case presentation, and differential diagnosis. Obviously, the goal of the ICM sequence is not to produce a fully formed clinician but rather to lay the ground work for clinical attitudes and skills that the student will be expected to build on during the 3rd and 4th years.

All of the ICM courses are taught in small groups or seminars. The faculty/student ratio is low, from two to eight students per faculty member, depending on the course. Many faculty members from a variety of disciplines volunteer their time to this course resulting in a contribution of approximately 5,000 teaching man hours per academic year.

The interviewing course which we teach meets for 2 hours weekly during the Winter and Spring quarters of the 1st year. During the course, four students are assigned to a physician preceptor who accompanies the students to nearby hospital in-patient services where students conduct interviews with hospitalized patients. After the interviews, the students get together with their preceptor and discuss the experience in depth. Students also have the option, during the course, of videotaping some of their interviews.

* * * *

Increasingly, in medical publications and in the lay press, one hears words such as "humanism", "wholism", and "holistic." It is not always clear precisely what these words are meant to convey, and different authors seem to use them differently. What is clear, however, is that many people, from many different viewpoints, are beginning to realize that something is seriously wrong with medicine—something that goes beyond the soaring costs of health care, beyond problems of health care distribution, beyond the awesome technical complexities of contemporary practice. It seems to many people that an essential respect for the human spirit itself is increasingly disappearing from medicine.

Traditionally, medical education, particularly in the first 2 years, has paid little attention to the humanness of the student or his patient. Clinical attitudes and skills are assumed to materialize at the appropriate time, as though trained empathy will automatically appear when the student begins his first clinical rotations in the third year. The fact that ICM courses are being integrated into the core curricula of medical schools nationwide attests to a growing appreciation that, while empathy and human aptitude must begin with native talent, they can also be developed in a fertile climate. Conversely, in a destructive educational setting, these qualities can be stifled, if not destroyed.

Hence, the title of our book—Patient Interviewing: The Human Dimension. We believe that this book represents a solid introduction to the techniques of medical interviewing, but it is our hope that beyond this, a spirit informs the book which exults the joy of our humanness. This has been, and always will be, the essence of medical practice in its highest form.

This book begins in Part I with an attempt to understand the experience of becoming a physician and the experience of becoming a patient. The first chapter is a story about a student and the relationship he formed with one of his first patients. It is not a transcript of an interview. Rather it depicts what the initial process of the relationship between student and patient is really about—what each of them brings to it, how each of them interacts, and how each feels, experiences, and ultimately grows from involvement with the other. In Chapters 2 and 3, we will describe the experience of becoming a physician and that of becoming a patient. In Chapter 4, illness will be viewed as a developmental crisis containing common stages through which each patient must pass. We will discuss the factors which may enhance successful resolution and those that can impede it. The influence of the physician in this process will be considered.

Having set the tone of the student-patient encounter in Part I, in Part II we will focus more specifically on the interview itself. We will cover common issues which students and patients cope with prior to the interview, during their encounter with each other, and (an important and neglected area) after the interview. We will cover some common ways in which students and patients tend to get fouled up with each other during the interview process—not simply through misapplications of technique, but in emergent problems in the way students and patients are seeing each other during the process of their encounter.

Finally, in Part III, we will consider the medical history. In Chapter 8, we will explicate its components and discuss the medical write-up. In Chapter 9, we will turn our attention to the art of obtaining a good medical history.

Often clinicians find that the shift from an open-ended stance with their patients to a more directive one feels awkward and abrupt. In this chapter, we will emphasize an approach to history-taking that builds upon the doctor-patient alliance rather than disrupting it. We will show how it is possible to obtain a content-directed history in a way that is integrated with a stance that permits continued receptiveness and empathy for the patient as a person. In Chapter 10, we will examine three actual interviews that illustrate how content and process, directiveness and receptiveness can be successfully combined.

Because no book can be effective if it simply explicates concepts in a vacuum, we will introduce these concepts as they arise in actual clinical material that demonstrates interactions between patients and students rather than "expert" interviewers. We will use many clinical vignettes derived from our experience as clinicians and teachers to illustrate appropriate points. Naturally, in order to protect confidentiality, the names of all doctors, students, and patients have been changed.

Our purpose will not be to show examples of "good" and "bad" interviewing techniques, for each student must ultimately develop his own style. There can be guidelines but no rigid rules or nostrums. We will cover the "nuts and bolts" of interviewing—the technical issues and factual content of interviewing technique thoroughly. We will do so, however, in the context of the doctor-patient relationship. For it is our conviction that these principles will have much greater meaning to the student when they are developed within the context of an appreciation for the rich, lively, *human* process that unfolds when doctor meets patient.

The book is designed primarily for beginning medical students who are learning to work with patients for the first time. We believe that the book can serve as an appropriate text for interviewing courses which are part of an ICM sequence. Beyond this, we believe that the book will be of value to more advanced physicians who are interested in deepening their understanding of the interview process and the richness of the doctor-patient relationship. Since a variety of non-M.D. professionals have intense, daily, life-long contact with the medically ill, we also believe that the book is a useful reference for nursing students, clergymen, social work students, and other individuals whose work brings them into close contact with the medically ill. Above all, we have written this book for those professionals within our ranks who believe that the ultimate responsibility, and joy, of our profession lies not simply in the acquisition of scientific knowledge and technical skills but also in sharing with our patients in the rich, often dramatic, always fascinating, human drama that unfolds when we work with a person who has turned to us for help when he has fallen ill.

D.E.R.
A.K.S.

ACKNOWLEDGMENTS

Throughout the writing of this book we have been especially indebted to three individuals: Dr. Richard C. Simons, Ms. Pat Riddle, and Ms. Salvinija Kernaghan. Dr. Simons, beyond reading extensive portions of the manuscripts and offering very helpful suggestions, was an inspiration throughout. His encouragement and faith in the ideas that we have tried to convey in this book have been invaluable. The lion's share of typing for the manuscript was done by Ms. Riddle who cheerfully and unbegrudgingly turned out draft after draft. Beyond her contribution as a typist, in itself monumental, she approached the project with great insight and understanding and thus has contributed substantively to the final product. Ms. Kernaghan, our editor, did a magnificent job of polishing and tightening the final product—she accomplished this by understanding not merely the letter of the book, but its spirit.

We are grateful to the following individuals who reviewed portions of the manuscript and offered helpful suggestions: Dr. Steven Dubovsky, Dr. Kathleen Gresh, Ms. Bridget Milnes, Dr. George Mizner, Dr. Emily Mumford, Dr. Calvern Narcisi, Dr. Fredric Platt, Dr. Jean Robinson, Dr. Michael Solomon, and Dr. Curtis Stine.

Although the following individuals did not directly review the manuscript itself, their contribution as senior colleagues to our own understanding of the educational process has been great: Dr. William Bernstein, Dr. Douglas Carter, Dr. Homer Olsen, and Dr. Herbert Schlesinger.

For helpful suggestions regarding the title of the book, we would like to thank Dr. Patrick Roney.

Additional valuable secretarial support was provided by Ms. Vicki Black, Ms. Josie McHugh, Ms. Janice Quintana, and Ms. Elise Stone.

We are grateful to Mr. Norman Fringer for lending us his dictating equipment for over a year without complaint or threat of an overdue notice.

We are greatly indebted to our editors at Williams and Wilkins, Ms. Toni Tracy and Ms. Alice Reid. Their patience and support have gone far beyond the line of duty.

Over the years we have read many acknowledgments in textbooks wherein the authors thank their families for general encouragement and support.

Before we wrote this book, we did not appreciate how great their sacrifice really is and how critical their support turns out to be. Thus, for all the late night hours, manuscript pages cluttering the kitchen table, and panicky searches for dictating cassettes lost behind the toaster, our deepest thanks for your patience—and our deepest love. Finally, to the many students and patients who contributed to this book—some of whom actually appear in these pages, all of whom have left their mark—we owe our deepest respect and gratitude.

D.E.R.
A.K.S.

CONTENTS

part I

DOCTORS AND THEIR PATIENTS

chapter 1

THE FIRST PATIENT

September 25, 6:45 a.m.

In an hour, Paul Stevens will meet his first patient. The course is called "Freshman Interviewing—An Introduction to the Doctor-Patient Relationship." The title of the course does not describe Paul's feelings, however, for although he has been in classes for 3 weeks, this morning will be his first time up on the wards of the hospital. In the dim light he pushes aside the cup of coffee he had made himself. It is already growing cold. He has barely touched it, for he is nervous, though he doesn't like to admit this to himself. He tells himself instead that this morning is really no big deal. He's only going to go *talk* to a patient. And he has talked to people all of his life. Yet, doubts surface. What if the patient is silent and Paul can't get him to talk? Or hostile? Or even crazy? He heard that *that* happened to one of his classmates earlier in the week. A thousand "what if's" run through his mind.

He goes into the bedroom and straightens his tie in front of the mirror. He puts on the white coat he bought at the bookstore yesterday and then pins his new name tag over the left breast pocket. It takes several tries to get the tag lined up straight. He notices that the price tag is still dangling from the lapel of the coat and cuts it off with his wife's manicure scissors.

As far as Paul is concerned, he still doesn't look like a doctor. With his new Litman stethoscope in one pocket and a thick manual of lab values and procedures in the other, he should look like a real doctor, but he feels like an impostor. The coat isn't part of him. Wearing it like this makes him feel like he's pretending, and this makes him uncomfortable. The day before, Paul argued this very point in class. He was among those who argued that students wearing white coats and calling themselves doctors is an exploitation of patients—that they are subtly "lying" to their patients, poor people in a county hospital being used for training purposes. He still feels this way; but this morning in the pale light, he simply thinks to himself, "This isn't me."

His preceptor will be Dr. Irving Gellman. He hasn't met Gellman yet.

The word from the sophomores is that he's OK, "a nice guy," one student
told Paul. Whatever that means, Paul thought. Paul received word the day
before through Gellman's secretary to meet on Ward Six North at 7:30 a.m.
Dr. Gellman had to meet with the students early so that he could attend to
his own patients across town on rounds later that morning.

Paul shrugs his shoulders and turns from the mirror toward his wife Joan
who still lies nestled enviably in sleep, the sheets pulled up over her head.
He kisses her lightly and whispers good-bye. They have been married less
than a year. They moved from St. Petersburg, Florida, so that Paul could go
to medical school in Los Angeles. He is 22 and she is 21. Being a year behind
him, she had to drop out of college after her junior year. The plan is for her
to go back and finish her senior year at UCLA "as soon as possible." For
the moment, however, she is working to help put Paul through medical
school. At 9:00 she will drive to the medical center herself in the old VW
(their only car) where she works as a secretary in Radiology. This morning
Paul will ride in on his bicycle. He locks the door behind him and ventures
out into the smoggy L.A. morning. At 7:15 he chains his bicycle to a fence
near the medical school. Across the street the County Hospital scowls down
at him through the smog like a massive concrete magistrate. It is the largest
building for miles, and it dominates the east L.A. landscape. Paul was told
by one of the sophomores that the building had once been used in a movie
version of Orwell's *1984*—The Ministry of Information. Paul can believe it,
for it is huge, impervious, and seemingly indestructible. During the Depression, it held many thousands of patients. In more recent years, the census
has been reduced to a little more than 2000, but it remains one of the largest
hospitals in the country. Paul has heard other doubtless apocryphal stories
about the building: that its walls are 3 feet of solid granite and so strong they
could not be dented by the wrecker's ball, and that deep in its bowels, its
foundation rests on huge iron rollers which could withstand any earthquake.
It is as though people regard the building as a symbol for illness and human
suffering itself, eternal and, in the end, indefeatable. Paul looks up at its
myriad windows. So many sick people in there, he thinks.

* * * *

He entered through the basement and weaved his way down the corridors
toward the elevators that went to Six North. The basement itself was a
fascinating labyrinth of intense activity. All around him people hurried this
way and that. They all seemed to have one thing in common, in contrast to
Paul: they knew what they were up to and where they were headed. Young
men in white linen uniforms drove electric tractors that towed huge carts
full of linen along the corridors. Kitchen workers pushed stainless steel racks
brimming with plates that contained the patients' breakfasts. Messengers
scurried everywhere. Nurses walked briskly on their way to work. Every so
often Paul saw an intern or resident, distinguished by his surgical greens (as
opposed to Paul's crisp white jacket), drooping eyelids, and, it seemed to
Paul, a certain unmistakable self-assured and knowing look.

A group of these interns and residents clustered a few feet from Paul waiting for the elevator. At their center stood a graying man with a long white coat, their attending. They talked loudly, competing with each other for his attention. Despite the presence of many nonmedical people waiting for the elevator—including visitors as well as ambulatory patients—they freely discussed "the liver failure on Four North." Oblivious to everyone outside their circle, they chatted eagerly about a particular lab value and how it related to an article in the *New England Journal of Medicine.* The gray-haired man seemed impressed.

So was Paul. Looking at these three men and two women, in their authentically crumpled surgical greens, Paul felt very acutely the gap between himself and these "real doctors." Although their rudeness in talking about the intimate details of a patient in front of visitors had not eluded him, he envied their self-assurance. By contrast, he felt like a complete bumbler. Once, during a brief tour of the wards when he first arrived at medical school, he had seen young men and women like these conducting a cardiac resuscitation. They had functioned so smoothly, with such aplomb. Paul had been terrified and had stood at the doorway, half in and half out. And just the day before he had struggled unsuccessfully to draw 5 cc of blood from his lab partner during a practice session. How would he ever be able to run a resuscitation?

Up on the sixth floor, he was innundated by sights and sounds that were new to him, unfamiliar musky smells, strange equipment, tubes, monitors, bottles, and i.v. poles. He couldn't help gawking at one patient, literally half a person. (Paul had heard of this operation, a hemicorporectomy, but it was very different seeing its results and what they really meant.) There, as alive as Paul, was a young man about his age, chopped off at the trunk. He wheeled himself about vigorously on a gurney. His big biceps bulged under rolled up sleeves, and he wore a tatoo that said "Hell raiser." With a scraggly beard and unkempt long blond hair, he looked a lot like patients Paul had seen at the free clinic where he volunteered. Except this one had been cut in half. Yet there he was chatting, actually flirting with a couple of nurses in the hall who giggled in response. Paul felt ashamed of his desire to stare. He upbraided himself for having "morbid curiosity" and tried to turn away and act more "doctorly."

He was again struck by the almost regal confidence that the interns and residents on the floor seemed to emanate. They moved in clusters, chatting, sipping coffee from styrofoam cups. He heard a bellboy go off. "Doctor Jordan . . . Doctor Jordan . . . call extension 7482." Though these young men and women were actually little older than Paul, really only students themselves, they struck him as being light years ahead in maturity and experience. As he approached Six North, he passed another gurney where a frail, wrinkled old woman lay on her back. She was clutching a brown paper sack with her name written on it in pencil. She was wheezing heavily, obviously having trouble getting enough air, and clearly in pain. Paul could see, even with his untrained eye, that her lips were cyanide blue. Was this the difference his professor had been talking about in lecture when he referred to "pink puffers" and "blue bloaters"? Somehow this old woman seemed like much more to Paul than simply a "blue bloater." He was tempted to stop and do something for her, but he didn't know what; besides, she wasn't even his patient, he told himself. So he went on.

By the time he found Gellman and the three other students who were part of his interviewing group, it was 7:30. And Paul, who had come through the doors of the hospital barely 10 minutes earlier, already felt tired, over-stimulated, and bombarded with a thousand new sights, sounds, and emotions.

Gellman seemed reasonable enough. He had fashionably long hair and a mustache. He wore cords. All of this put Paul at ease, for he had feared that Gellman might be one of those formidable professors in long white coats. Gellman had a wafer thin bellboy clipped to his shirt pocket. Paul saw this for the status symbol it was. He had already noticed that in the hierarchy of the medical pecking order, less is more. The interns trudged around with big bellboys sagging from their belts, pockets laden with pamphlets and examining equipment. Residents often dressed in street clothes and usually carried only a stethoscope stuck in their hip pocket. Attendings, like Dr. Gellman, wore no equipment at all, except for the wafer thin bellboy.

"I've got a great case for you," Dr. Gellman said to Paul. "Leukemia. Acute lymphoblastic leukemia." They agreed that for this first interview, the other students would go off and interview their patients on their own. This morning Gellman would go with Paul. In the coming weeks he would rotate through to observe the other students.

"Her name is Mrs. Clark," Dr. Gellman added, almost as an afterthought.

He grabbed a chart from the rack in the nurses station and led Paul in to see his first patient. Paul ran through in his mind the steps he was to take in the interview, the steps he had read, the steps he had been lectured about the day before. Establish rapport. Make eye contact. Ask simple questions. Identify yourself to the patient. But somehow, in spite of himself, all of these considerations were far from his mind when he first laid eyes on Mrs. Clark.

Sitting up expectantly, alone in a room with three other empty beds, Paul saw a smiling, emaciated black woman who had no hair. Yet, there she sat, in a pink bathrobe, holding in one hand a Holy Bible and in the other a mirror and a brush. She saw Paul staring, first at her bald head and then down at the hand which held the brush. She then looked down at the brush herself and with a smile and flustered apology said, "I forget sometimes, first thing in the morning."

Despite how thin she was, her face was broad with high strong cheekbones. She had large expressive brown eyes and a full-lipped engaging smile. Her face was the kind that invited trust even in strangers, and her expression said, "Don't be afraid, come closer." Despite her baldness, her demeanor was unmistakably feminine.

Paul took a second to gain his composure.

"Good morning Mrs. Clark," he finally said. "I am Dr. Stevens."

He had been encouraged by Dr. Gellman to introduce himself that way, but having said it he immediately felt like a complete phony. He hastily added that he was "a student doctor." Then, . . . "A freshman." Mrs. Clark smiled, nodded, and waited expectantly.

Paul then muffed his opening line. He had been told in lecture to ask, "What sort of troubles have you been having?" Instead he repeated himself, nervously introducing himself a second time as "Paul Stevens . . . Dr. Stevens . . . a student doctor." Once again Mrs. Clark smiled and waited.

"Ah, um, how are you, that is?" Paul stuttered.

"I'm fine," she said patiently.

"Um, I see . . . um . . . "

She seemed to empathize with Paul's discomfort, for as he stammered and fidgeted she leaned forward toward him and raised her eyebrows encouragingly, as though she wished to help him, like a fledgling actor, over these difficult opening lines.

After a bit more fumbling, Paul managed to find himself a chair and to seat himself by the side of her bed. He tugged once on the knot of his tie, cleared his throat, and began to try to sound "doctorly."

"What sort of troubles have you been having?" he finally remembered.

She said succinctly, "I have leukemia."

At this point Paul was dumbfounded again and didn't know what else to ask. Mrs. Clark helped him.

"I have a form of leukemia called acute lymphoblastic leukemia," she said. "The doctor first noticed it when I came down with a bad sore throat. Plus, I'd been experiencing a lot of fatigue. They're treating me now with chemotherapy." She gestured toward her i.v. line. "That's what this is for."

"Oh," said Paul. "I see, that stuff is for the canc . . . that is for the, ah, leukemia?"

If his almost saying the unspeakable—that dreaded word "cancer"— bothered Mrs. Clark, she gave no sign of it. But Paul felt sick inside. What had he said? What damage had he done? He turned to Dr. Gellman, who stood silently at a distance, but Dr. Gellman had not seemed to react either. He was busy flipping through the lab data in Mrs. Clark's chart.

Despite the awkward beginning, the two of them soon began to hit it off. She told Paul she was eager to talk with him and had been looking forward to meeting him since the nurses had told her the day before that a medical student would be coming to see her.

"It's always nice to have visitors," she said cheerfully.

Paul began to feel more at ease.

He learned that her disease was relatively rare in black people. That was why at first her doctor had thought it must be something else, a bad anemia, or maybe, because her liver was enlarged, an unusual case of hepatitis; but she said in the end there had been no doubt.

Mrs. Clark was 36. With obvious pride, she told him that she was already a grandmother. She had a 6-month-old granddaughter, her daughter's child, and they lived in Ventura County, not far from L.A. Mrs. Clark said cheerily that her daughter came to visit her "often." In fact, she said, she had many relatives out here, though her family was originally from Baton Rouge, Louisiana. Brothers and sisters, many cousins. They, too, came to see her "often." All the same, in the coming months, when Paul would come to visit with her, he never saw anyone joining her in the empty room. In fact, for some reason that he did not understand, since all of the houseofficers were constantly carping about the high census, no patients ever seemed to be placed in any of the other three beds during Mrs. Clark's hospitalization—that is, with the exception of one old woman in her 80s, transferred from a nursing home in terminal congestive heart failure, who died within 2 days. Mrs. Clark admitted to Paul that sometimes not having a roommate made her feel lonely.

"Maybe they think I've got the plague or something," she tried to joke.

Mrs. Clark was a widow. Her husband had been a career officer in the Army and she spoke of him with obvious love and pride. She reached into her purse at one point and showed Paul his picture—a smiling handsome black man in a Captain's uniform. She told Paul that he had been shot down in Vietnam.

Throughout the interview, Mrs. Clark hacked and coughed. Paul didn't want to tire her and asked her several times if she wished to stop the interview, but she would shake her head emphatically and say, "No, that's fine." She explained to him that the drugs she was taking to attack her leukemia also lowered her resistance to infection. The cough, she said, was due to "a little case of pneumonia."

In spite of her "many visitors," she told Paul that she enjoyed very much the chance to talk to a young doctor. She had several nice young doctors and mentioned two of them by name. But they were very busy and seldom had a chance to talk. At one point in her animated, cheery discussion, while she was speaking proudly of her new granddaughter, she reached out and touched Paul's hand. Paul experienced a feeling of warmth, but then began to worry. Was it wrong to touch a patient's hand?

What seemed to bother Mrs. Clark the most—more than her pain, more than her cough, more than the knowledge that she had leukemia—was the fact that she was bald. "I'll bet a good-looking young doctor like you has better things to do than spend time with an ugly old lady like me, sitting here bald as you please, bald as a bed post," she joked halfheartedly.

"Oh, no," Paul protested. "It doesn't look bad at all."

Weak, he thought to himself; that was a *weak* response. There must be a better one, he thought, but he didn't know what it would be so he responded to her in the best way he knew how. "You don't look ugly to me at all, Mrs. Clark." He meant it.

"You're just saying that, doctor," she said, but smiled all the same. She told him her hair loss was due to one of the drugs that was being used to treat her leukemia, called vincristine. With a sigh, she supposed that such a side effect was worth getting "the best medical treatment you doctors can provide." The drug also caused shooting pain in her arms and legs and occasionally some numbness, but this didn't bother her too much. Her deep faith in the good Lord helped her when there was pain. If only she weren't so vain, she laughed. "You caught me with the brush this morning. It's just that when I first wake up each morning, sometimes I forget—well, no . . . that's not true. The truth is that sometimes I *pretend*. I say to myself, 'Today I'll look in the mirror and I'll be a beautiful young woman again . . .'" She laughed. "I hope that doesn't make you think I'm crazy, doctor. But it's just that at one time I really wasn't bad looking—for a grandmother; that's not boasting, just the truth. And these changes," she said, "these changes are hard to accept. Sometime I'll show you a picture of what I looked like when I had my hair."

Paul's attention had become so riveted on Mrs. Clark that he felt oblivious to his surroundings. He had forgotten about Dr. Gellman in the background, and even the rest of the room had become a blur. He was engrossed. Moreover, he found himself responding easily, naturally. He felt as though he were being himself. Yet, he was very aware that, as she talked to him, she was treating him as though he were her doctor. It felt good.

He was feeling so good, in fact, that he did not notice the arrival of the respiratory therapist, until suddenly he was being elbowed aside by a scowling middle-aged black woman who was shoving a plastic green mask over his patient's mouth, even as Mrs. Clark was speaking. "Respiratory therapy now," the intruder barked. "She's got to have her mist now." "Move your chair—No! No! Back. There, out of the way. Can't you see the machine here!"

Paul felt furious, helpless, and humiliated all at once. In the hospital pecking order, freshman medical students obviously did not rank high. He also felt in a bind. He sensed that it would be demoralizing to both himself and his patient to let this rude intrusion go by unchallenged. Yet, the idea of "pulling rank" didn't seem very dignified either.

He turned awkwardly to Dr. Gellman for help. For a moment, Gellman just stood there, smiling what seemed to Paul to be a subtle but unmistakably wry smile. Then Gellman stepped forward. It was Paul's impression that the respiratory therapist had not noticed Gellman initially because he stood in the background.

"Come back here," he snapped at the woman. "This doctor and I are examining this patient. You will have to come back later. Do that thing later."

The therapist stared at her opponent. Her eyes narrowed and she bit her lower lip pensively. Sizing the situation up, she heaved a sigh, glared at Gellman, and yanked the mask from Mrs. Clark's face. Lugging the machine behind her, she muttered under her breath, "I've got my job around here, too."

Paul felt extremely uncomfortable, even disgusted. For one thing, coming from St. Petersburg, he was very sensitive to the racial overtones of the situation. What meaning would it have to his patient, a black woman, to have witnessed two white doctors backing another black woman down? Above all, though he felt as if his wish were naive, he wondered why people in the hospital couldn't work together for the good of the patient. During the confrontation, Mrs. Clark had been little more than a human sack of potatoes being bandied about in the battle of her caretakers' egos. He didn't know which felt better, being pushed around or doing the pushing. In any event, Dr. Gellman used the opportunity of a break in the interview to invite Paul to examine Mrs. Clark with him. He had been looking through her chart and told Paul that her case showed some "interesting findings." In particular, he wanted Paul to feel her enlarged liver.

He invited Mrs. Clark to recline, which she did without protest. Although Dr. Gellman's voice was gentle, Paul noticed that he had not introduced himself to her first. Dr. Gellman carefully pulled the bed sheet up just over her hips and then lifted her hospital gown up just below her breasts, baring her abdomen.

"Relax now," he said, "and take a deep breath."

Mrs. Clark obeyed. When she exhaled, Dr. Gellman placed the fingers of his left hand under her rib cage and his right hand on top of his left.

"Now take a deep breath."

She began to breathe in, and as she did so Dr. Gellman plunged his fingers up into her rib cage. Paul saw her grimace but she voiced no discomfort. She continued to inhale and suddenly Gellman smiled and nodded.

"Here," he said to Paul. "I'll show you."

He guided Paul's hands onto her abdomen. Several tries . . . Paul could feel nothing. He wanted to quit. He had just begun to feel some mastery in his role as a student doctor when he was talking to Mrs. Clark. Now he was forced to be a novice again, trying to feel her liver, and he didn't like it. And he was worried about subjecting his patient to excessive discomfort. Gellman, however, insisted that he persist.

"You'll never get it if you don't stick with it. You'll know it when you feel it. It'll feel like something coming down and brushing over the tips of your fingers."

Paul nodded and asked Mrs. Clark to breathe in once more. This time he pushed his fingers deep into her rib cage and sure enough, something firm and rubbery brushed across his finger tips, like a fish surfacing from the deep. He was so delighted that he broke into a broad smile, almost a laugh of excitement and triumph. He was no longer attuned to the increasingly fatigued, pained expression on his patient's face as she repeatedly underwent this procedure. Dr. Gellman and Paul then tried to feel her spleen because one intern had reported in her chart that it was enlarged; but they were unable to feel anything and concluded that the intern had "a healthy imagination," as Dr. Gellman put it.

Dr. Gellman finished by showing Paul some enlarged lymph nodes in Mrs. Clark's neck. Then he told her that they would have to stop. Mrs. Clark asked if she could pull her gown back down, for she had obediently left it where Dr. Gellman had placed it over her rib cage during the examination. Dr. Gellman said, "Of course." Mrs. Clark then smiled and said, "Thank you very much, doctors." Somehow this sounded odd to Paul, especially after all the poking and prodding they had done—as Paul saw it, only for his benefit. It felt like an exploitation, and yet here she was *thanking* him. He in turn found himself saying enthusiastically, "Thank *you*, Mrs. Clark." Somehow that sounded awkward to him too, but he wanted to say something. Then he added, gratuitously, "You've been a great patient." And immediately he regretted saying something that sounded fatuous.

Afterwards Dr. Gellman and Paul and the three other students met in a conference room to talk about their cases. Paul had half expected Gellman to light into him, especially since Paul felt he had "blown" the interview from a technical standpoint. He presented his case to his peers with animation, obvious involvement, and enthusiasm, but he was highly critical of himself nonetheless: he had forgotten to ask open-ended questions; he had talked too much at points; and he had forgotten to repeat the last words that the patient said, the way he had read he was "supposed to." And then there was the business of whether or not he should have held her hand. And he had not closed the interview properly or summed up at the end the way he should have. It seemed as though everything he was supposed to do, he had forgotten.

Dr. Gellman smiled and nodded. He agreed with Paul that he had forgotten to do a number of those things.

"But all the same," he asked, "how'd you *feel* about the interview?"

Paul hesitated and said, "Well, to be honest, I think I *did* come across insecure, but I really thought she was interesting." Then he added more assertively, "And I think she liked me."

"So do I," said Dr. Gellman. "And that's important. You had a nice way with her."

Paul beamed. Toward the end of the discussion Paul commented in passing that it would be nice if he could somehow follow up on what happened to her. How could he find out who her doctor was and call him?

"Why don't you follow her yourself?" Dr. Gellman suggested.

Taken aback, Paul said, "Who me?"

"Why not?" Dr. Gellman asked.

"Because . . . uh . . . " Paul did not go on. He had been about to say, "I am not really a doctor. What do I have to offer?" But he didn't say it.

"One thing you should keep in mind," Gellman said. "You might really become important to her."

Paul nodded and unconsciously began drumming his fingers on his knee.

That night he excitedly tried to share his experience with his wife Joan over dinner. She tried to listen attentively at first, but she also wanted to tell Paul about *her* day. Paul reacted by feeling that she wasn't really interested in what he was telling her and rather smugly implied that she probably "can't really understand." Joan then barked at him crossly. "All you ever talk about anymore is medicine. Sometimes these days you act like one big medical machine. Your increasing narrowness these days slays me, Paul."

This hurt him, and it worried him too, for he knew that he had become increasingly obsessed with his courses; he was aware of how consuming his studies had become, how narrow his interests and repertoire of ideas were growing. One night not long before, at a party for students and their spouses, he had suddenly realized that all he talked about the entire evening was neutrophils and the Krebs cycle. And this did alarm Paul. For he felt the gap widening between him and Joan for the first time. And beyond this, really, he felt a gap widening between what he was becoming and what he had been. True, he had been a premed major in college, but he had minored in English Literature and had taken the minor seriously. Now it seemed, the only poetry he recited was mnemonics: "On Old Olympus' Towering Top . . . "

Yet, tonight at dinner he wasn't talking about neutrophils. He was saying something very important to him, something about the most *human* thing that had happened to him since he had started medical school. A patient! His patient! And it made him sad and cross that Joan seemed vaguely envious of his enthusiasm and either could not or would not understand.

But, then again, Joan had been increasingly moody for weeks. At times she would be excessively clinging, demanding repeated reassurances from Paul that he loved her. Sometimes on these occasions, when he was studying at the dining room table, she would plunk herself down in his lap and demand kisses and hugs before she would let him return to his studies. At other times she would be uncharacteristically cross and hypercritical, making fun of Paul and his classmates for being "drones" and "zombies." A proud, highly intelligent person, Joan had been elected to Phi Beta Kappa in her junior year, before dropping out to go West with Paul, but now she was always accusing herself of being "purposeless and dumb." On one occasion, when a recipe for chicken overcooked, she had cried inconsolably for hours saying, "I'm dumb, stupid, worthless. Why don't you get rid of me?"

Not demonstrative by nature, and inherently somewhat uncomfortable with strong emotions, Paul had tried to think of ways to solve Joan's problem. Why didn't she join the Wives' Club? That she said was "nothing but a bunch of crap." Perhaps she needed to go back to St. Petersburg to visit her family. Maybe she missed them. Paul's own characteristic mode of solving problems was to act in some way, to do *something*. But whenever he proposed solutions, this simply seemed to upset Joan even more.

He told himself it would pass.

October 19, 9:00 a.m.

This particular morning in anatomy lab, Paul had a disturbing experience. In the weeks since their initial encounter, Paul had been meeting with Mrs. Clark at least once or twice a week and they had grown very close. He had come to enjoy her warm gentle laugh and her endless stories of ancestors and relatives who dated back to the time of slavery. Occasionally he worried about her, especially during one period when she went into what the resident told him was a "blastic crisis" and had to be transfused; but even when she was quite sick he never thought much about the eventual inevitability of her death. She was simply too vibrant and alive. Moreover, he kept his involvement with her very separate in his mind from the rest of his medical school activities, the endless hours of drudgery, memorizing, microscope gazing, and dissecting that consumed his waking hours. When he thought of Mrs. Clark, she was the patient he was following in the hospital "across the street." This morning, however, as Paul and his lab partners began a dissection of their cadaver's hand, Paul was horrified to find that he kept thinking of Mrs. Clark's hand. He tried to put the thought out of his mind but, very uncharacteristic for him, found himself unable to do so. He became anxious and distracted. Looking across the lab to another table where four students were engaged in a dissection of the abdomen, he saw one of them reach into a cadaver's belly and pull up a large clump of small intestine and mesentary. With a chill, and very much in spite of himself, he imagined Mrs. Clark lying on a slab in the autopsy room, her belly split open, the pathologist pulling out and scrutinizing her intestines. Finally Paul got so upset that he left the lab early. Fretfully, he asked his wife Joan that night, "Am I going crazy?"

Thursday, October 21, 8:00 p.m.

Every Thursday evening, Paul got together for a 3-hour session with his "study group," a loose coalition of three other students and himself. Though they did get some studying done in these sessions, primarily during grilling sessions where they would quiz each other on trivia from the previous week's course material, the group also served an important social function. They would consume endless cups of hot black coffee, puff self-importantly on cigars, and talk animatedly about a variety of subjects during their "study breaks." Sometimes they would just gripe, sometimes philosophize. Often they simply shared.

Tonight, Paul had something on his mind. "Seriously," he asked. "Was I crazy?" He described in detail his anxiety attack in the anatomy lab earlier that week. His friend Gordon shook his head and stared at Paul with a quizzical, blank expression. No, nothing like that had ever happened to *him*. Paul really did begin to think then that he was crazy. But after a while, Richard spoke up. He had been reluctant to share this with anyone before, but from the beginning of the term, whenever he worked on his elderly male cadaver, he had thought about his grandfather who had died the year before. He had even developed a fondness for the cadaver and had given him a secret name, Harry, which had been his grandfather's name. Richard had decided in the loneliness of his own secrecy that that was "so damned sick" that he wasn't going to tell anyone and probably wouldn't have had Paul not disclosed his experience with Mrs. Clark.

John, who had sat in silence puffing intently on his cigar, then confessed that sometimes when he worked on his cadaver he had a recurrent thought that he couldn't get out of his mind. His cadaver was a female. Over and over, he would find himself thinking, "this could be my wife . . . "

November 5, 6:00 p.m.

Paul had become quite busy with his studies. He had a practical coming up in Anatomy and in 2 weeks a midterm exam in Histology. He had told Mrs. Clark that he would see her around 4:00 the previous day but had gotten tied up. At 4:00 he had called the nurses' station and asked them to tell her he'd be over at 4:00 the next day instead. By the time he got up to the floor, it was closer to 6:00. Also, because he had spent the day in the library, he went to visit her dressed in a pair of slacks and an open-neck shirt. On all previous occasions, he had worn his white coat.

In recent weeks, Paul had noticed that Mrs. Clark had become increasingly sensitive to his arrival time. Although she never complained or expressed irritation, almost invariably she would comment if he arrived much later than he had promised. And he had been late more and more recently as his study load increased.

He found it hard to understand why this mattered so much to her since, as he saw it, he wasn't really that important in her treatment. He thought of himself as "really just her friend."

Tonight, though, something seemed to be bothering her. Finally, she began hesitantly, "Doctor, are you on vacation?"

"No," Paul said. "What made you think so?"

She hemmed and hawed.

"Well," she said, "it's probably silly, but, doctor, without your coat on you don't *look* like my doctor."

She said it with a pained, apologetic expression and hastened to add, "It's just a silliness of mine, an old-fashioned thing I guess."

"Did I ever tell you about my oldest brother?" she asked Paul.

"No," Paul said. "You've never mentioned him."

"Well," she said, "he was very important to me when I was growing up. In some ways he reminds me of you, doctor."

She went on somewhat wistfully to tell Paul a story that he had not heard before. When she was 6 years old, her father had died of a heart attack. Her oldest brother, Sam, was 16. He had been a sophomore in high school but had to drop out to support the family.

"My mother told him," Mrs. Clark said with a smile, "that now he was the man of the house and would have to take care of all of us women. For you see, there was my mother and me and three other sisters; but with Dad's death, that left Sam as the only man." She sighed. "He was very good to us. Sometimes I think he must have resented it, all those women hanging on his sleeve, I know I did, making demands on him that were pretty heavy for a 16-year-old boy. But, you know, he did all right. In the end, he really did all right. He turned into quite a man. He wanted to be a doctor. But as you know, at that time, for a black person to become a doctor was almost unheard of. And with Dad's death, it became impossible. But he was able later to go back to school and now he's a physical therapist."

"In many ways," she smiled, "Sam and you are a lot alike."

Later that night in the library, where Paul was in the habit of studying, he was thoughtful. Through one of the library windows he could look across the street up at the big county hospital where Mrs. Clark lay. The white coat thing bothered him a bit. It had been Paul who had argued so vocally that wearing white coats was a kind of deception and exploitation of patients. Yet Mrs. Clark had made it very plain to him that his white coat was far from an exploitation. Like it or not, she *expected* Paul to be her doctor. Whether he felt ready or not. Maybe some of his ambivalence about the white coat had been his own discomfort with being seen as a doctor. In any case, he found himself musing about the stories she had told him of her brother Sam, who had to assume great responsibility whether he felt ready for it or not. At some level, had she been saying something to Paul about *his* importance to her as well?

November 18, 10:00 a.m.

It was a brisk Fall Saturday morning, one of those rare days when L.A. was free of smog and one could see all the way to the San Gabriel Mountains. Paul and Joan were preparing to go on a car camping trip, their first weekend together not consumed by his studies since he had begun medical school. The phone rang. It was the hospital operator. She apologized to Paul for calling. In fact, she stated somewhat officiously that she was not actually allowed to call people about patients unless they were really doctors. But one of his patients was sobbing uncontrollably and refused to talk to anybody but Dr. Stevens.

Giving his disgruntled, perplexed wife a peck on the cheek, Paul headed for the door, promising that he'd "be back soon."

When Paul arrived at the hospital he found Mrs. Clark alone, trembling in her bed, sobbing openly. It was the first—indeed the only—time he would ever see her cry. When she saw him at the doorway, she stretched her arms out to him and pleaded with him silently to come to her. At this point, Paul's instincts guided him. He went over to the bed and held her in his arms. He had no book to tell him to do this. Dr. Gellman was not there to guide him. In fact, he wondered if he was doing the right thing, sitting there on a bed, hugging his patient who sobbed in his arms. But he did it anyway. Paul, the master problem solver, simply had to let his feelings guide him. On this occasion, like many others that would come in the future, there would be no one to guide him and he would have to do what felt right.

Eventually, the story came out. Mrs. Clark was in another severe blastic crisis, receiving many transfusions. A new medical intern had told her that afternoon that she was "terminal" and probably had "less than a couple of months" to live. It hurt Paul to see how distraught this had made her. She had said to him many times before that she knew her illness was "terminal." But now that he thought about it, she had never actually said, "I'm going to die." And now she sobbed in his arms and repeated over and over, "I'm going to die. I just can't believe it. I'm really going to die. I had such a *life* ahead of me! So much left to do! It's not *fair!*"

And then Paul saw her do something he never thought he would see. She picked up the Bible that lay on her bedside, slammed it onto the floor, and shouted, "Goddamn it! Goddamn it!" She flung it with such force that the i.v. bottle tottered on its pole and then crashed to the floor causing a nurse to come running. "Goddamn *that* too!" she shouted.

And then, to Paul, "You're all I've got, doctor, you're all I've got."

Later Paul went to the nurses' station in a fury looking for "the lousy _____" who had been so blunt with his patient. But when he found "the lousy _____," he turned out to be a slender, well meaning young man named Walter, just out of medical school himself, who was doing his first rotation on internal medicine. Walter earnestly quoted to Paul from a book by Elisabeth Kübler-Ross about the need for honesty with "the dying patient." Paul thought to himself, "This isn't exactly the dying patient—this is Mrs. Clark!" But somehow Paul sensed that Walter, in his own way, was really no different from himself. He too was stumbling through new stresses and responsibilities of almost unimaginable magnitude, with little help or guidance, in the end basically on his own, doing the best he knew how. This insight calmed Paul, but it also disturbed him. For with it came an important bit of self-knowledge. He realized that he had derived some previously unacknowledged security from looking up to the interns and residents as being all wise. They weren't.

And, it should be added, by the time Paul got home it was 2:30 in the afternoon. Their plans for a weekend of camping had been dampened, if not ruined, and Joan didn't know whether to take him in her arms, or let him have it, or both.

November 21, 7:30 p.m.

Joan walked into the bedroom and found Paul lying on his back, wearing only his jockey shorts. He had both hands dug deeply under his rib cage and was staring up at the ceiling, taking deep breaths.

Joan: Paul, what in the world are you doing?!

Paul: Checking my liver. I think it may be enlarged. (Sitting up in bed, he pulled down his lower eyelid to expose the white of his eye.) Come here a minute, Joan, take a look at this. Does my eye look a little icteric to you? A little jaundiced?

Joan: Oh, Paul, for heaven's sake. For the last month you've been "catching" every disease you read about. (Then, her expression softened) Sometimes it must be scary for you. Seeing all that. Knowing all that. Sometimes it must be really scary.

December 2, 3:00 p.m.

A day of triumph! Mrs. Clark's wig had arrived. Paul had personally and single-handedly triumphed over the usually intransigent hospital bureaucracy by persuading someone in Central Supply that a wig was essential to Mrs. Clark's medical well being. As wigs go it wasn't much. At least it was brown, since he had specified that it was for a black woman, but it was cheaply constructed of synthetic fibers and clearly styled for a Caucasian woman. Still, when Mrs. Clark put it on, they both reveled gleefully. How beautiful she looked! Paul had done this for his patient, Paul and no one else. It was a deeply meaningful moment for him. In some crazy way, he thought to himself, conning a wig out of Central Supply had put him one step closer to being a real doctor.

Mid-December

Toward the end of her life, Mrs. Clark began to experience much more pain and was rapidly losing weight. She was on heavy doses of narcotics and often would simply ask Paul to hold her hand while she dozed. She was very tired. When she was awake, she would speak quietly and wistfully of her past life and accomplishments. There was one thing happening about that time of which she was especially proud. In the spring, her youngest daughter would enter college, a small Catholic girls' college for blacks in Baton Rouge. She had lived to see every one of her children college educated.

She also talked more about her brother, Sam, the older brother who reminded her of Paul. For the first time she told Paul that Sam had recently died. About 8 months before, he had been fatally and tragically shot in Louisiana in a love triangle. Mrs. Clark had been grief-stricken. A month later, she was diagnosed as having leukemia. Although, as she said, "It doesn't make any sense really," she had a funny feeling she just couldn't shake that *somehow* the loss of her brother had brought on her leukemia.

Paul knew that the end was approaching. He had gotten to know some of the housestaff by then and a lot of the nurses. He taped a big sign to the front of Mrs. Clark's chart which read: "Please call Paul Stevens, medical student, *night or day* in the event that Mrs. Clark is terminal."

December 21, 2:45 a.m.

Paul was awakened out of a deep sleep by the phone ringing on the bedside stand.

"Are you Paul Stevens, the medical student? I saw your note on the front of Mrs. Clark's chart. You probably ought to get down here. She's "corred" out twice in the last 3 hours. They're working on her now."

December 21, 3:30 a.m.

Paul ran down the hallway to Six North and rushed into her room, his heart pounding. He expected to see a half dozen people working feverishly over her. Instead, to his shock, the room was dark, empty, and absolutely still. For a minute he wondered if the phone call had been a dream. There was Mrs. Clark's bed. Empty. It had already been freshly made with crisp new linens. The bedside drawer that had held her possessions was empty, its bare metal drawers hung open. Like metal tongues, Paul thought, awaiting pills. The window at the far end of the room had been pulled open and a slight breeze wafted through the darkened room.

In a rare efficiency that the County Hospital reserved only for death, Mrs. Clark's body had already been trundled off to the hospital morgue. Housekeeping had been called and the room had been cleansed, the bed remade. At 3:30 in the morning!

Then, under the bed, Paul saw something that chilled and sickened him. There, crumpled up, forgotten, was her wig. Probably it had fallen off during the resuscitation and been overlooked there. With trembling hands he bent down and picked it up. He brushed it off. His lips began to quiver with grief and rage.

How could they?! How could they take her down there to the morgue and not even have the decency to give her her wig?! Then he realized what an idle, almost silly thought this was.

It was over. There would be no more visits with Mrs. Clark, the proud, smiling black woman from Baton Rouge who had become his first patient. He lay the wig down on the bed and just stood there for a few minutes, thinking, reminiscing. Paul finally got up and left the room. Out on the ward, a wall clock read 4:00 a.m. The ward was silent except for the sound of a respirator in a nearby room. Every few seconds there would be a click, then a sound something like air rushing from the nozzle of a tire. The lights in the main corridor had been dimmed. Down at the far end of the hall, one dusty window framed a pale, wafer thin moon. It's wan, tepid light fell like a thin mist on the roof tops of nearby buildings in the medical complex. Beyond them, Paul could see the Santa Ana Freeway, headlights crisscrossing in a racy confusion, even at this time of night. Life goes on. One intern sat hunched over the counter in the nurses' station, writing a note in a chart. Two nurses sat chatting quietly. The nurses' station was the only place on the floor that was brightly lit. Through the metal and glass, the intern and the two nurses looked almost surreal, like a television picture with the brightness turned up too high.

As Paul passed, one of the nurses came to the doorway and motioned to him.

"Are you Paul Stevens?" she asked. "The medical student who was Mrs. Clark's friend?"

Paul nodded.

"I'm Mrs. Brady," she said. "I'm the nurse who called you earlier."

"Thank you for remembering me," he said.

She was an elderly woman, with graying hair. She wore her nursing school cap, a rarity among the nursing staff since they had done away with the requirement a few years back.

"We haven't met," she said, "because I'm on permanent nights. But I have read your notes in the chart."

That's unusual in itself, Paul thought to himself. For awhile he had written notes that were quite lengthy, but as time went on they became short and at times nonexistent, because he honestly believed that no one read them.

"I have something for you," Mrs. Brady said. She reached into a drawer and handed Paul a bulging envelope. In Mrs. Clark's handwriting—neat, feminine, and small—it said, "For Dr. Stevens." "She gave this to me about a week ago," the nurse said. She made me promise that I wouldn't give it to you until after her death. So here it is."

With trembling hands, Paul took the envelope and walked quickly to a vacant stairwell down the hall.

He sat down on the steps. Inside the envelope was a small silver caduceus and a letter. The letter read:

Dear Doctor Stevens,

I can never fully thank you for what you have given me. I have often marvelled at how you found the time for just one patient like me. I am sure you have others and I know how busy your days and nights are with all the studying you must do. I know you will be a better doctor for it, but I want to thank you especially for the time you found to spend with me.

I am not a philosopher, that's for sure, but I think I've learned some things about life, especially here in the hospital with me having leukemia and all. As I'm sure you know, there are many empty hours and a lot of time to think. Sometimes I must confess that I do think about dying. I hope you will forgive me if that sounds morbid. I guess it is a little, but my faith in the good Lord is very strong and somehow I feel it is important to think about these things, at least some.

My father died when I was a little girl. My husband died tragically 5 years ago. As I recently told you, my big brother died just 8 months ago and in many ways that was the hardest death to take of all.

I guess the point that I'm trying to make is, for all of that, knowing the reality of death doesn't make you that much more prepared for your own. I have always been very afraid of dying, and still am, though I know in my heart that the good Lord will always take care of me. But there's something I figured out recently that I wanted to share with you because I think it's important for you to know this if you're going to be the fine doctor for your future patients that you have been for me. And that is, that the worst part of dying is the loneliness. For a long time I could not understand why my relatives, especially my daughter, never seemed to come to visit me. I never really admitted this to you, doctor, probably because I had trouble admitting it to myself. But they really didn't come around as often as I said and deep down I was hurt and mad. But I think when you're dying, people forget about you. Maybe it's that they're scared or don't know what to say, but it almost feels to me like they've grieved me and forgotten me before I've finished being alive and before I've grieved myself!

Anyway, that's where you come in. You have been a most wonderful doctor to me and a most wonderful friend! You never let me down, and like I say, I know that must have been hard with your schedule and with me just being one patient and all among so many. I cannot tell you, doctor, how much this has meant except to say that you have been very important and very dear to me. I hope you will not misunderstand what I mean if I tell you that I love you. I think you will understand.

This caduceus belonged to my father. He was a pharmacist, one of the first black pharmacists in the South. Although I was too young to know him well, I have been told that he was a great, wise, caring man—like you. My mother gave this to him when he graduated. It's made of real silver so be careful not to lose it! I am giving it to you because you have meant so much to me and because I wanted to give you something very, very special and important to me. I guess I'm also giving it to you because I hope in the years to come you will sometimes think of me and remember me.

This has been kind of a sad letter and I'll stop now because I know we have many times yet ahead to talk with each other and I look forward so much to all of our conversations! But I did want to get some of this down in writing and to tell you how much the time you have spent with me has meant. With deep affection and appreciation,
    Adele C. Clark

He did not fight the tears back any longer . . .

After what seemed a long time, Paul carefully refolded the letter and returned it to its envelope. He put the caduceus in his pocket and walked slowly down the stairwell to the first floor of the hospital.

On his way out he ran into Mike Simmons, an internal medicine resident whom he had gotten to know when he had been rotating up on Six North. Mike had been one of the doctors who had taken care of Mrs. Clark over the months. Sometimes, it had been hard for Paul to keep track of them for house staff seemed to come and go without warning. But Paul had particularly respected and liked Mike.

"How's it going, Paul?" Mike asked, with a big smile as he hurried on his way somewhere.

"Do you remember Mrs. Clark? The lady with leukemia on Six North?" Paul asked.

"Sure," Mike said. "How's she doing?"

"Well," Paul said, "she died this morning."

Mike nodded. There was a moment of silence.

"How are things going for you overall?" he finally asked Paul.

"Well," Paul said, "I'm getting there."

"Slowly, but surely," he said "I'm getting there."

He walked out into the still, blue morning.

chapter 2

BECOMING A DOCTOR

A central premise of this book is that becoming a doctor is a developmental process, a crucible of emotionally intense experiences that most medical students undergo without adequate recognition or help. Almost all of medical education focuses on the student's acquisition of technical knowledge and skills (the content) at the expense of attention to the changes he is undergoing (the process). I believe that this onesidedness ultimately dehumanizes the experience for student and patient alike.

Recent changes in medical school curricula suggest a positive trend, however. Especially, the increase in *Introduction to Clinical Medicine* (ICM) courses throughout the country signals greater awareness of the importance of early, meaningful exposure to patient care in the student's education. Nevertheless, medical education still has a long way to go; it remains monolithic and tradition-bound in many respects—ultimately conservative and wary of change, often more preoccupied with the histology of tissues than the potentialities of people.

Thus, I deliberately begin this chapter with a description of one of medical education's oldest institutions, the dissection of the cadaver. I believe that the student's early exposure to the cadaver is not simply an introduction to important medical content but is, in a curious way, a metaphor for much of the education that will follow. The process of dissecting the cadaver turns out to be, in my view, at least as important for the student as the content knowledge that the experience imparts.

THE CADAVER

During the spring of his freshman year, Dan had the following nightmare:

He was at a party for his medical school class. The party was being held in the evening in the anatomy lab. Although this was obviously an inappropriate place to be having a party, no one seemed to notice or mind the presence of numerous cadavers. Indeed, the lab was festooned cheerfully with pink crepe paper and all of the students were laughing and joking and seemed to be having a good time.

Dan became increasingly frightened, and then he panicked. He was afraid of the cadavers. He tried to tell his close friend, and roommate, about his fears, but the roommate brushed him off with the comment that he was being too sensitive.

At that point, to Dan's horror, one of the cadavers lurched up into a sitting position and pointed an angry finger in his direction. Dan started to run from the room...

He woke up in a cold sweat.

As Knight has observed, medical school traditionally begins with the dissection of a cadaver. This is probably not accidental because the student's relationship to this first patient becomes a powerful symbol for much of what follows in the course of his professional training.

Dan's dream highlights many important issues that face every medical student: the fear of death, guilt over violating the tabooed sanctum of the dead, and some deep-seated universal fears about how little separates the living from the dead. Perhaps most revealing is Dan's own understanding of his dream. Naturally introspective, Dan lay awake for a half-hour after the dream woke him and pondered what it meant.

"What really disturbed me about it," Dan said, "was the inappropriateness of it. Here we were partying in the anatomy lab. It was like we had all become so callous—we could even have fun in a morgue."

Dan felt he was changing in ways he didn't fully understand and certainly hadn't expected. He found himself wondering to what extent his life had become synonymous with an all-consuming preoccupation with disease and death.

"That's what I think the party stood for in the dream," Dan said. It meant something like, here we all are, getting our jollies in life out of things like disease process and cadavers. I've really changed. We've all really changed. I'm not sure I like it!"

Initiation Into the Guild

Beyond the cadaver's importance for introducing the student to anatomy, its dissection early in the first year of training represents an important rite of passage into an exclusive and mysterious guild.

Scott was speaking excitedly to an old college roommate during the Christmas break of his freshman year of medical school. His roommate had entered graduate school in accounting.

"What's it like?" his old roommate asked. "I mean what's it *really* like to work on all those dead people?"

Scott had tried to downplay things. "You get used to it," he had said. "It's just part of learning about the human body."

Underneath, Scott had been uncomfortably aware, however, of the authority he had suddenly acquired in his friend's eyes. Somehow, the fact that he had dissected a cadaver set him apart, made him special, and perhaps just a little awesome to his friend.

The dissection of the cadaver sets the student apart symbolically from the rest of society. Typically, the student experiences this as lonely, yet exhilarating. He is a doctor; his right to dissect dead people is one of the first and most potent symbols that he is different.

Denial of Death

The cadaver is a silent, yet blunt and unrelenting reminder that death confronts us all. Compared to physicians, most people enjoy considerably more denial in their daily lives.

Consider the phenomenon of a highway accident. Traffic slows to a crawl. People drive by slowly, staring at the sight in stunned silence. They are suddenly and unexpectedly confronted with the reality of death. It is a profound jolt—soon to be forgotten.

By contrast, the medical student quickly learns that he cannot regularly enjoy the luxury of ignoring this reality. Beginning with the cadaver and continuing into his clinical work with the sick and dying, the medical student is constantly reminded of his own mortality and the mortality of those he loves. How he copes with this has a great deal to do with the ultimate shape and flexibility of his professional identity.

L. L. Stephens described the experience this way:

> The study of medicine is in fact the study of living and dying. No more central nor enormous concern seems to exist, or at least this seems so for the peculiar and puzzling species of men and women who elect to take upon themselves the role of physician. And the innermost mystery of all, the most frightening, the most compellingly interesting, the most inescapable truth encountered in this journey is that one cannot learn about living and dying only in others. One cannot help but make inferences about one's own life and death ... it seems true beyond doubt that upon comprehension of living and dying depends ones ability to serve as a physician.

The Myth of Finite Knowledge

Dissecting a cadaver also explodes the myth that medical knowledge, though vast, is ultimately masterable with enough hard work. No student entering training nowadays is naive enough to believe that medicine is a static, unambiguous body of knowledge. Every student knows that his training will require learning prodigious amounts of new facts. Still, students may harbor the understandable wish that, with increasing knowledge, they will achieve greater security, not further uncertainty. In fact, increasing knowledge in medicine brings both.

Yet, students are often quite unprepared for the impact of medicine's ultimate ambiguity and uncertainty. They enter medical training sharing the biases of our culture. Although today's public is better informed about medicine, especially its problems, people continue to cherish a deep wish that doctors know everything and that they be able to apply this knowledge effectively to treat disease and cure it.

All cultures need to see their healers as absolute authorities. This phenomenon is most apparent in so-called "primitive" societies. However, the scientific revolution has done nothing fundamental to reduce these magical expectations in Western cultures. The only difference is that now our Western expectations are more subtle, yet, ironically, more demanding. While healers in primitive societies can invoke religious and mystical explanations for their failures, our contemporary society's reverence for the new religion of science demands far greater perfection from the physician.

The entering medical student is a product of this culture and naturally, although not always consciously, shares its expectations. At some level, almost every medical student hopes that medical knowledge will be doled out in its entirety, over 4 years, in serial fashion, like issues of an encyclopedia.

Physicians generally have a strong desire that medical science be exact and finite for other reasons as well. There is good evidence that those of us who are attracted to medicine are frightened by illness, abhor helplessness, and resist loss of control. Many doctors place a high value on order, thoroughness, and exactness in the conduct of their lives. Deep down, many physicians hope, "If I work hard enough, study long enough, learn everything I possibly can, then my own feelings of vulnerability, frailty, and uncertainty will be mastered."

Initially, the cadaver seems to hold out an enticing promise of meeting these expectations. Anatomy is one of medicine's oldest and most thoroughly explored disciplines. The cadaver itself appears vastly complicated, yet ultimately concrete, comprehensible, and finite. As the student progresses in his dissection, however, it begins to dawn on him that, even in anatomy, our knowledge is far from complete.

One freshman medical student expressed mild shock when he found out that every vein in the body is not named. "*Gray's Anatomy* is almost 1500 pages of fine print!" he exclaimed. "Surely they'd have named all the veins!"

Of course, all the veins cannot be named. Individual variation is too great. Variations in many organ systems are so common that there really is no norm; the anatomy of the biliary ducts is an example. And certainly the experience of dissecting the human brain underscores our present ignorance about mental functioning. Cognition can hardly be explained by the masses of nondescript glial cells that one sees swimming under the microscope.

Finally, on the most pragmatic level, students soon find that, no matter how many hours of study they put in, there is always some question that their anatomy teacher comes up with on a test that they cannot possibly answer.

Thus, the cadaver, at first so invitingly inert and unchanging, turns out to be a symbol of considerable uncertainty and lack of closure. In its own silent way, the cadaver demands that the student face up to ambiguity; and it makes this demand of individuals who, by and large, find ambiguity unnerving. The cadaver is an early and powerful symbol of our ultimate helplessness, not only over death, but also over ignorance.

Learning to Dissociate Thoughts From Feelings

In his work with his cadaver, the student also learns one of medicine's most important yet dangerous lessons; namely, that by dissociating one's thoughts from one's feelings and one's intellect from one's emotions, one can do almost anything.

Some students may have seen a corpse before they entered medical school. A surprising number have not. In either case, as students anticipate the experience, it stimulates a mixture of excitement and dread. They are about to behold a dead person. They will cut into it—into its heart, its brains, its genitals. It was once a human being, yet now it is dead and will be unable to protest. The experience is new, often awesome, and even mystical. What is perhaps more surprising, however, is how quickly students cease to be aware of feeling anxious at all.

A few weeks into anatomy, students regularly adjust. They become used to probing into body cavities of dead people. The cadaver quickly ceases to be a dead person, at least as far as the student is aware, and becomes instead an object of study and memorization. Only occasionally do students experience conscious recurrences of the old dread and awe that they once felt in the presence of the dead.

Most of the time, after the first critical incisions, the only signs students give of any further uneasiness about their sojourn into the land of the dead will be found in a tendency toward gallows humor and some surprisingly resilient and long-lived mythology that makes its way into the lab. For instance, there is the story about the students who chopped off the arm of their cadaver, handed it to a toll keeper, quarter and all, and then drove away leaving him clasping the disembodied arm. This story has probably been told in most medical schools in the country. One wonders, in fact, whether the story doesn't say something about where our submerged feelings go. Could it be that by traumatizing the patsy in the toll booth, the medical students inflict on him the anxieties they once felt themselves but soon forgot?

When a casual visitor drops in on the anatomy lab, what he beholds are clusters of students grouped around tables, reading from books, grilling each other on anatomical trivia, intent on concentrating, certainly not emotionally aroused. What he is witnessing is the sight of students who have mastered one of medicines most powerful tools, the ability to evoke intellect before feelings and to convert feelings into ideas, then to manipulate these ideas, and finally, at times, to forget the original feelings that once underlay the ideas.

It is quite amazing, in fact, to observe the rapidity with which feelings go underground. Within the first 2 years of medical school, students will have learned not only how to slice into dead people but also how to undress and penetrate living people.

This defense is absolutely essential for the effective learning and practice of medicine. The problem for most students, at least at certain points in their training, is the defense's surprising power. Many students who enter medicine valuing their capacity to feel find it disconcerting to discover how facile they become about cutting off those very feelings. To do so seems essential. The surgeon could not operate without this ability. Yet, it makes many students feel a bit like Doctor Jekyll and Mr. Hyde. Once one learns to cut himself off from his feelings, it is sometimes frightening to realize how difficult it seems to get back in touch with them. This cannot always be done at 5:00 p.m. on schedule, and the student soon learns, like Dr. Jekyll, that the potion doesn't always wear off when it's time to go home.

The Cadaver As Patient

Another phenomenon that we sometimes see during the dissection of the cadaver is the development of a distorted perception of what the doctor's "ideal" patient should be like. The cadaver can leave the physician longing for similar attributes in his later living patient. Our first patient is silent. He does not protest. He demands no attention, no reassurance, and he never fights back. With this patient, the doctor is always right. Or if he isn't, his patient never says so. Some doctors do in fact seem to get angry at their difficult living patients because they do not display the passive, uncomplaining qualities of their first dead patient.

Obviously, this model of the doctor-patient relationship is limited. It is a model in which the doctor acts upon his patient, who in turn receives his actions passively. Although it certainly represents one aspect of the doctor-patient relationship—the most obvious example is surgery—there are other models of interaction that are as important in medicine. One is the model of mutual collaboration, in which the patient is seen as an active participant and collaborator with the doctor in the process of his treatment. The cadaver obviously has a very limited contribution to make here.

"Science" versus "Humanism"

One might ask whether I am focusing too much on the symbolism of the cadaver to the exclusion of its obvious practical value. Yet, ultimately I am not questioning the need for learning gross anatomy, or even its timing in the curriculum, though I do think the latter has some hidden significance. I am asking why the aspects of this experience that are so symbolically loaded, so emotionally intense for the student, have been so widely minimized and ignored. In the instance of the cadaver, as in so many situations in medicine, the real question is not whether students need to be exposed, but rather how we can help them experience the exposure as growth promoting rather than traumatic. To do so, in my view, requires us to consider students' feelings as well as their intellect.

Why then have we traditionally placed the cadaver so prominently at the beginning of the student's journey—unless to signify its importance as a rite of passage, a kind of ritual hazing? Could this not unintentionally denigrate the real value that dissection can have for the physician? Certainly, its timing cannot be justified on the basis of clinical relevance; students have always complained that they have forgotten much of the anatomy they memorized by the time they begin their clinical rotations several years later.

My contention would be that the cadaver's symbolic presence at the beginning of the student's education imparts a different message: it promotes in students' minds the dichotomization of medicine into two polarized, seemingly irreconcilable factions: The "humanistic" versus the "scientific."

For many students, facing their first cadaver presents them with a cruel choice. If they acknowledge their anxieties about what it means to dissect a dead person, they are not up to the task of being detached and scientific, as medicine seemingly demands. Yet, if they stifle these very real feelings in themselves, they have become "scientific" at the expense of their own feelings, indeed their own sense of humanness. This dichotomy is rife throughout various stages of medical training. It is as dangerous as it is silent. The cadaver is the first of many situations in which the student, mistakenly feels that he must choose between being objective and scientific on the one hand or sensitive and humane on the other. The goal of medical education should be the integration of these concepts, not their polarization.

I recall my own experience as a freshman medical student in the anatomy lab. One day, a group of orthopaedic residents joined the class. With great intensity and concentration, they dissected a cadaver's hip. When I asked what they were doing, the residents explained that they were practicing to do a hip operation on one of their living patients the following day. Here was a group of more experienced physicians, allowing the dead to help them improve their skills for the living. It epitomized the very best of medicine's ideals and exemplified medicine's real potential for integrating the scientific with the humanistic. Far too often, medical education seems instead to promote a false division between the two.

THE EXPERIENCE OF CHANGE

There is a useful though imperfect analogy between the development of the physician and the indoctrination of the medicine man in primitive cultures. Here is an excerpt from Kenneth Keniston's excellent article, The Medical Student:

> In primitive societies, those who would become shamans or witch doctors must often undergo curious rites of passage. At an early age, the future shaman is frequently set apart from others by his conviction that he possesses special healing powers, which may be transmitted by virtue of his birth into a healing clan; from the start, his fellow tribesmen endow him with a special mana of one who will confront the ultimate mysteries of life and death. On reaching maturity, and perhaps after enduring ritual ordeals to test his vocation, he is apprenticed to the elders whose ranks he will join. Often he is secluded from his fellows for many years, submitting to painful initiations to establish and consolidate his calling. In these years the secrets and stigmata of his guild are passed on to him—frequently an arcane language, dating from the distant tribal past, a special manner of relating himself to the sick and to the dying, and an elaborate technology of herbs, charms and incantations to preserve the living or hasten the dead upon their way. Upon emerging from his prolonged initiation, the young shaman may be expected to assume a new name, to don the distinctive garb and amulets of his order, and to accept the ambivalent weight of membership in this feared and powerful guild.

This very evocative analogy raises many issues pertinent to medical students. It articulates powerfully the fact that the goal of medical education is to change students. Change is not a side effect of the educational process but its goal. There are other lines of work in which this is not true; one can learn to be an airline mechanic, for instance, without changing fundamentally as a person. This is not the case for a doctor. He learns a skill, to be sure, but he is also transformed as a person.

Change is never an unambivalent experience. For most of us, the new is sensed as dangerous until familiarity proves it otherwise. To change involves not only the acquisition of new skills and competence but also the loss of a sense of connectedness to what we used to be. Therefore, it is not uncommon that medical students, along with the excitement that accompanies their growth, also experience some degree of mourning for the old selves they leave behind.

> Roger had been an anthropology minor in college with a major in premed. Several months into his freshman year of medical school, he brought a number of anthropology books into his laboratory space and put them on the shelf next to the texts of anatomy and histology. Another student had asked with some vexation what a textbook on primate social behavior could conceivably have to do with the histology of kidneys. Roger, almost offhandedly remarked, "Oh, I don't really think I'll read it—it's just nice to have up there to remind me who I was."

At best, change will be experienced as traumatic as well as exciting, a touch painful, and sometimes a little sad. We do not relinquish our old selves without some grief and protest. Often, however, the process of change is experienced by medical students as more traumatic than it need be. This may be because the student receives very little help during his formal education in developing rational, flexible ways of coping with the changes he experiences. One very obvious instance of this is the drastic change most students experience from the preclinical to the clinical years. The philosophy seems to be, "sink or swim." Most students do eventually learn to swim. A few sink. Do they sink because they were made out of poorer quality stuff? Or does our educational system fail to help them? And of the far greater majority who swim, how many end up more hobbled by the experience than they need to be?

To take but one example, one of the enduring ironies of the medical education process is the disparity between the way students and houseofficers are treated and the way they are expected to treat their patients. Residents are expected to be up all night, every third night, sleep in grubby call rooms, and then be grilled the next morning by their attendings on bits of medical minutiae. Is it logical to expect that people treated this callously are then going to be able to treat their patients any differently?

Typically, students become aware of the fact that they are changing in two phases. First, the student realizes that people in his environment are treating him differently; usually this change becomes quickly apparent during the first months of medical school. Though it is disconcerting, this phase of recognition is usually not as painful as the second phase, during which the student begins to realize that he has changed not only in the eyes of his environment, but also in his own.

The Experience of External Change

It takes only one cocktail party during which the student is "consulted" by one of the guests to make him aware that he is changing in his relationship to the rest of the world. Similarly, it takes only one trip home to visit family, where the student is met by admiring yet uncomprehending responses from his relatives and old friends, to underscore the loneliness of this new and special role he has decided to adopt.

Estrangement from family can be especially painful. Separating from one's family of origin and establishing a distinct identity is a major developmental task for people in their 20s. How different persons achieve this task can be quite variable. Some individuals find it easier, at least for a time, to repudiate everything their parents represent. This sometimes makes cutting the umbilicus easier, and reconciliation a few years later is common. For such individuals, entrance into medical school may provide a welcome opportunity to set themselves apart.

A great many other students in their 20s, however, retain close ties to their families and wish to reduce but not obliterate their sense of connectedness to their families. For these students, their parents' lack of real comprehension regarding what their children are doing can be painful. In addition, such students are often disconcerted to find that their parents, whom they always looked up to, are suddenly deferring in subtle ways to their son or daughter now that he or she has become a "doctor."

Don was an energetic and creative sophomore with a talent for basic research. He described his disappointment about his return to Cleveland one Easter vacation and his attempt to share his excitement with his parents. His mother was a housewife. His father ran a small but successful hardware business. Both were very proud of him.

"They were pleased for me, and proud of me," Don said. "I knew that. But beyond that, I looked in their eyes and saw I was drawing a blank. I tried to explain to them the special project I was doing in immunology. They said, 'That's great.' And they meant it, but they had no awareness of its significance or importance—to them it was just all part of the same blur—I was their son, the doctor."

The experience of external change can also be difficult for married students. Sometimes students come to find that an invisible yet impenetrable wedge of incomprehension, and even jealousy, has grown between husband and wife.

Ann was a junior medical student when her marriage began to feel the strain. Her husband, Tom, a teacher, told her he was thinking about having an affair with someone at work. Ann was shocked and hurt.

For the first 2 years of medical school, they had been close. In spite of her great academic abilities, Ann had only been accepted to one medical school out of the many to which she had applied. This was in a crowded, smog-infested city that neither Ann nor Tom liked. During those first years they had been united in a common struggle—the smog, the urban decay, and the drudgery of hassling with the different bureaucracies each faced.

Then, in her junior year, Ann came alive with excitement. After her initial anxiety, she found that she loved her work on the wards. She achieved great success. One of her attendings told her that she might get nominated for Alpha Omega Alpha during her junior year. When Ann tried to share this with Tom, he had stared at her coldly.

"You know," he said with a steely edge in his voice, "I never thought you'd change so much as to get excited about something as mickey mouse as some student honor society." A short time later, he told her he was contemplating an affair.

The Experience of Internal Change

The second phase of awareness of change, during which the student begins to feel cut off not only from friends and relatives but also from his former self, occurs early in medical training and typically accelerates during the clinical years. The awareness becomes more intense as the student more and more successfully adapts to his new role of physician; indeed the sense of inner change is a by-product of that mastery.

The experience is described by Keniston:

> There are moments in the life of every medical student when he awakens suddenly to realize that he is no longer reacting emotionally to events, experiences, and activities that would once have terrified, shamed, or upset him deeply. For a few, such realization may be unequivocally positive; but for many, relief and triumph are mixed with concern lest in some way the student is becoming depersonalized, automatized, mechanized, or in some other way losing his capacity for ordinary human responsiveness. It is as if, especially during the first years of medical school, the students were frightened lest defenses elicited and strengthened by medical school were to spread, cancer like, into all areas of his life. Among students who have long prided themselves on their detachment, there is least to lose; but among those who pride themselves upon their sensitivity, sympathy, and openness to their feelings, to observe in themselves an *absence* of anxiety, revulsion, or fear could be surprisingly distressing.
>
> Thus it happens that many students wonder what medical education is doing to their humanity, their sensitivity, and their capacity for feeling. Among groups of first year medical students meeting to discuss the effects on them of medical school, the question "Are they leaving the human race?" recurs regularly and even monotonously.

Identity Panic

As students become increasingly aware of their isolation, from friends and relatives and their old selves, they may experience an identity panic. During this period, common worries include their perception that they have become arrogant and emotionally cold, too narrow as people, too constricted in their interests. Many students worry that their creativity has disappeared and been replaced by an obsession with medicine. It is no wonder, such students assert, that they are isolated. They feel they have lost their ability to relate to anyone other than fellow medical students.

It is not uncommon during this period to find students suddenly enrolling in art courses, taking up new hobbies, subscribing to concert series, and in extreme cases deciding to drop out of school in an attempt to combat their narrowness. Often students will try to broaden social contacts and renew old ones.

What students feel to be at stake is their sense of identity; the new hobbies, the art courses, are viewed as attempts to recapture highly valued parts of themselves which they fear they have lost. These attempts at self broadening do occasionally help. More often, however, the student feels disappointed. First, his free time is limited. He does not have the luxury of cultivating numerous new relationships or hobbies. More important, the quality of the time he spends with friends is important, and the wish for understanding is great. Therefore, students tend to stick with one another, not only for convenience and not simply because they are "in a rut," but because other medical students are often the most reliable source of support and understanding.

Adapting

Student advisors and counselors often give the same advice that students give to themselves: "Go out and make new friends, broaden your interests, take up a hobby, etc." Although this advice is not entirely without value, it is too simple. The student's identity panic stems from his real perception that he is changing inside. Attempts to graft on new activities and friendships will by themselves not do much to mute the experience. It is usually more helpful to acknowledge that important change is indeed occurring. This can be intrinsically reassuring. It is also helpful to provide students with opportunities to share their feelings; it is often very heartening to realize that one is not alone in a dilemma.

With time, students find that they generally do reintegrate valued aspects of their former "nonmedical" selves. What seemed lost forever turns out only to have been temporarily inaccessible. Exposure to physicians who have achieved some balance in their lives can be helpful. The potential for ICM courses here is great. Hopefully, in the relationships that students form with their preceptors, they will have a chance to see role models who have mastered some of these issues and can share their personal experiences with their students.

Formal and Informal Groups

Often it is a doctor who can best understand another doctor. Students should not be excessively hard on themselves, therefore, when they find that most of their friendships form with fellow students. The worry about narrowness aside, a great deal that is supportive and growth promoting can come out of such friendships.

At the University of Colorado Medical Center, students spend much of their first 2 years in assigned laboratory spaces called "UTLs." Often informal groups spring up among students who are physically clustered together in this manner. Each section of a UTL begins to take on its own life, developing its own rules, jokes, and history. The bonds, though informal and often expressed through humor, can be intense.

These students are not simply engaged in bull sessions. Rather these informal networks help students support each other through the turmoil of change. Lack of such support is one overlooked reason why students so often experience the beginning of their clinical rotations as traumatic. In addition to their greatly increased patient responsibilities, students also feel isolated, torn away from the informal support groups they had developed during the basic science years. A group of this type was formed by Paul and his friends in Chapter 1. This "study group" did much more than study. Its members supported each other through the process of change.

One might ask, therefore, why more effort isn't made to formalize such support groups. Why, for instance, are opportunities for medical students, interns, and residents to share their experiences with each other almost nonexistent? The party line states: No time—too busy! But probably a more fundamental reason is the deeper myth of the physician as lone soldier, the solitary hero who fights his battles alone, the Spartan who may bleed inwardly but never lets it show. This myth, in my view, is destructive, not only to the student's sense of well being but ultimately to patients. A doctor who believes that sharing feelings and seeking support is a "weakness" is apt to transmit this prejudice to his patients. How can such patients then be expected to open up and trust?

The small group teaching format of many ICM courses across the country represents an important preliminary step toward changing the notion that the strong doctor is one who stands alone and never turns to another person for support and understanding.

HUMAN LIMITATIONS AND VULNERABILITY

Limited Knowledge

Question: A great deal of what medical students learn in their formal scientific education will become outdated within a decade or two after graduation. True or False?
Answer: True.

Obviously, manifestly, and remorselessly true. The factual base in medicine has steadily changed in response to new findings about the nature of disease and the treatment of disease. The inevitable question that arises from such developments is whether any field of knowledge can change so widely and so consistently and still be called a science. An even more troubling question: How durable is medical education, if a substantial amount of what it taught has to be replaced regularly? Does the doctor become obsolete along with the outdated knowledge base?

The truth of this observation, stated here by Norman Cousins, quickly dawns on every medical student. It begins as early as the dissection of the cadaver. Later, in many different contexts, the student realizes that there are drastic limitations to the state of his knowledge—limitations of knowledge in the field and inevitable limitations in the student himself.

This recognition can be painful. Many students come to medicine with the hope that they will be introduced to a coherent body of knowledge that they will ultimately be able to master through diligence and then to apply with confidence. In the words of Knight, "The development of the ability to accept uncertainty and to deal with it effectively is for many students the most difficult adaptational task confronting them in medical school." This can be especially true for students whose temperment demands that they act, who have a predilection for intellectual mastery, and who prefer to use logic to reduce ambiguity in their lives to a minimum.

Further, to experience one's limitations is to experience vulnerability. This has implications for patients adjusting to illness as well as for students adapting to medical training, a similarity that I will discuss further in Chapter 4. It suffices here to note that many students acquire their motivation to become doctors partly from a wish to overcome their own sense of vulnerability. Often, in the childhood experience of doctors, one will find memories of personal vulnerability, some experience of frustration, terror, and helplessness brought on by illness in the physician as a child or in a parent or sibling. Such experiences can give students special empathy, but they may also lead to a childhood fantasy that persists into adult life, which goes something like this: "As a little kid I can't control what's happening to me, why I'm sick (or why my mother is sick); but when I grow up I'll be a doctor. Then I can control these things. I will be able to prevent them from ever happening again."

When such a wish collides with a student's growing awareness of his own limitations, the feelings of vulnerability and powerlessness can be distressing.

Personal Limitations

DOCTORS

They work with herbs
and penicillin.
They work with gentleness
and the scalpel.
They dig out the cancer,
close an incision
and say a prayer
to the poverty of the skin.
They are not Gods
though they would like to be;
they are only a human
trying to fix up a human.
Many humans die.
They die like the tender,
palpitating berries
in November.

But all along the doctors remember:
First do no harm.
They would kiss if it would heal.
It would not heal.
If the doctors cure
then the sun sees it.
If the doctors kill
then the earth hides it.
The doctors should fear arrogance
more than cardiac arrest.
If they are too proud,
and some are,
then they leave home on horseback
but God returns them on foot.

Anne Sexton

Each student must come to terms with his own personal limitations. The fact is, students are not all alike, nor will they be when they become doctors. The sheer vastness of medicine has promoted a trend toward specialization and subspecialization. As one academic physician, an individual with many publications on hepatic biochemistry, put it, "I'm a liver man."

This physician went on to say, quite candidly, that he knew he couldn't master everything, but he could "know everything there is to know about the liver." At one level, this reasoning is logical. It certainly provides patients with experts for almost every conceivable problem (at least if they are fortunate enough to be located close to a university medical center in a major urban area). On the other hand, specialization has tended to fragment medicine and fracture the continuity of patient care. The sad situation of a patient with a half a dozen specialists who doesn't know the name of his doctor is lamentably common. The current interest in a more holistic approach to medicine is a response to this.

Despecialization is probably not the answer to medicine's current problems. Specialization seems to be a necessary, inevitable response to the current knowledge explosion.

At the same time, students should anticipate the real allure of closing one's mind to certain types of experiences prematurely, out of anxieties over personal limitations. Some students have great gifts of memory that enable them to do well on basic science tests. Others have exceptional manual dexterity and thus may be spared the awkwardness that many students feel when they begin to do technical procedures. Still others have great natural capacities for empathy and can relate comfortably to patients in a clinical setting from the beginning.

Each type of student may at points be tempted to cope with his overall sense of limitations by channelling his aspirations and interests toward what he naturally does best. Thus, the empathically gifted student with a humanities background may assert, "I don't need to learn all that biochemistry, anyway. I'm going to be a psychiatrist." Similarly, everyone knows the would-be surgeon who, in his freshman year, has already picked out his residency and can't be bothered with patient interviews because "that isn't real medicine anyway."

Students who "specialize" prematurely as a defense are attempting to cope with a reality that medicine thrusts on all of us—we can't be perfect, we can't know everything. This can be an especially painful realization for men and women in their 20s. As Gail Sheehy has pointed out in *Passages*, the 20s are that period of life when people feel they can do anything; all it seemingly requires is hard work, endurance, and a faith in what one (secretly) believes are his own limitless capacities. According to Sheehy, most adults begin to reconcile themselves to their limitations during their 30s and 40s, when it begins to dawn on them that the choices they have been making have also been denials of other cherished wishes. Thus, the musically gifted pianist who becomes a corporate executive gradually realizes that he will never be a concert pianist, though he may continue to play for enjoyment.

By contrast, this normally gradual maturational insight dawns on medical students more abruptly, long before their 30s and 40s. Students quickly realize that there is too much to learn, that the field is too vast and bewildering in its dimensions ever to be mastered. For the many students who have considerable talents in areas quite removed from medicine, medical training can require some hard choices.

> John was a college track star with considerable talent in long distance running. Prior to medical school, he would begin each day by running 10 to 12 miles. In a number of AAU meets, he had finished with times that put him into the national standings. When he began medical school, his daily runs had to be shortened. First he tried to keep running 10 miles a day, then 5 miles every other day, then 2 miles as often as he could.
>
> "I just don't seem to have time to do everything," John said wistfully.

L. L. Stephens expressed the experience of human limitations and our need to come to terms with it this way:

> The work which we do is, in many respects, filled with impossibilities. Each of us is limited in intelligence, understanding, information, skill, sensitivity, and stamina. We have chosen to become physicians, among other reasons, because of some unusual attitudes toward responsibility. These attitudes do not always seem to me to be healthy. It seems to me that in our efforts to achieve excellence— which I believe should be unceasing—a proper sense of our limitations, a sense of humanity, of charity towards ourselves, are completely necessary qualities. To expect unrealistically of our teachers, of our peers, of our patients, and especially of ourselves, is to guarantee despair.

LOSS OF AUTONOMY

With the possible exception of the military, there are few experiences in a student's life that feel more restrictive and regimented than medical school. Many students feel especially constricted during the first 2 science years, but the feeling continues throughout medical school and into residency training. They are shocked by what they encounter in medical school after the experience of comparative freedom in undergraduate life. Students often find much of the lecture material inflexible, monotonous, devoid of creative thinking, and, as one student put it, "quite simply an insult to my intelligence."

Medical students find little room for electives. The message that clearly comes across to them is: memorize what you are told to memorize, learn the minutiae that we tell you to, and never mind asking questions about the point. In short, the student soon realizes that he must do as he is told.

Students also constantly hear, in countless subtle ways, that they know nothing and have nothing to offer. They are students, very much on the bottom of the medical pecking order. This, in turn, makes them feel uncomfortably dependent; their ignorance forces them to need the very professors they may also resent.

It seems almost diabolical that this experience should take place precisely at the point in many students' lives when they have finally begun to shake free of similar feelings from their own adolescence. It is difficult to generalize in this regard because many current students are older and more well established by the time they begin training. Still, most students enter medical school during their 20s, a period of life when they have recently separated from their families of origin and established their own identities.

Often college has served as a transition, during which students have relinquished the dependency of their adolescence and achieved increasing control over their own lives. This transition can be painful, and most people in their 20s at least periodically miss the security of adolescence and the safety of its proscriptions. For the most part, however, by the end of college, students are celebrating their freedom. They have mastered strong longings to return to the nest and have now turned their thoughts toward the future, wondering what they will carve out for themselves professionally, beginning to think about establishing intimate lasting ties with another person.

Thus, many students experience medical school as a forced regression, an unwelcome infantilization that they must nevertheless tolerate if they are to realize their dream of becoming doctors. As one student put it, "Let's face it—we're going to take whatever they dish out."

That students rebel at times is understandable.

REBELLION

At one medical school, during the turmoil of the late 1960s, a group of students decided to "decorate" their lab in defiance. Up went a large poster of a black radical cult hero sitting in a wicker chair, brandishing a spear and rifle. Other posters went up, quoting from Marx and Chairman Mao. The students decorated their desk space with the psychedelic posters so popular then.

Not surprisingly, some faculty reacted angrily. Some expressed concern that these students, who were sporting long hair and beads as well, were being unprofessional, refusing to "act like doctors." The long hair and beads that some students displayed up on the wards may have in fact disturbed some patients. By and large, however, the faculty was probably more distressed than were the patients. Some teachers felt frankly hurt, seeing in the students' behavior a rejection of what they believed in most and were trying to offer.

One famous ear surgeon, an older man in private practice, had for many years given an annual lecture to medical students on an operation he had perfected. This lecture had always been well received. Finally one year, facing an audience of bearded, long-haired, "revolutionary" students, he felt so hurt and offended that he refused to come back for the next 5 years to give his lecture. "These students don't give a damn about what I have to offer them," he had said. "So to hell with them!"

What was difficult for this teacher to appreciate was that, behind the abrasiveness, these students were trying as best they could to hang on to a sense of identity separate from their roles as medical students. One message inherent in their defiance was, "This is me, a part of me you can't regiment or control, something that is my own—my identity outside this place!"

The turmoil of the 60s gave way to a more quiet decade in the 70s. Not surprisingly, however, students today continue to express their wish for autonomy.

> One group of Jewish students from New York attending a Southern medical school, banded together and put a sign over their lab space reading "Little Manhattan." Their banter in the halls was often filled with Jewish ethnic references. Some professors, and other students as well, found their isolationism snobbish and insulting. Actually, these students were trying to preserve a sense of their own identity in the face of the erosion of individuality that medical school represented to them.

Students will sometimes complain about the narrowness of their curriculum and ask for electives and special lectures on topics of interest outside the traditional province of the curriculum such as acupuncture, home births, or herbs. Faculty should respect students when they request such material. Even if teachers feel at times that the material students are interested in is shallow, even bogus, students do have a right to some control over their intellectual fates. In this vein, giving students a meaningful role in various committees of the medical school is clearly a positive step. Students should be active participants on admissions, curriculum, and promotions committees and on other groups that determine medical school policy. These committees ultimately deal with the students' fate, and students should share the power of such groups.

RESPONSIBILITY

> Rich was a freshman when he had this experience:
> My wife and I were coming home from a movie. Up ahead we saw that there'd been an accident. A woman had been hit by a car. She was lying on the pavement and a crowd of people was standing around her. I felt my heart leap into my throat.
> My first reaction was, this isn't really happening. Then I heard myself saying,

"What's the difference, we can just drive on, the ambulance will be there soon anyway.

But then I realized, "You're a doctor! You *have* to stop!"

I tried desperately to remember what I knew. I raced through my mind trying to remember the details of the one lecture we had received on emergency first aid. We had received that lecture more than 6 months ago."

When Rich stopped, his worst fears were not confirmed. The woman had suffered a head injury but was conscious. She was reluctant to go to a hospital, and Rich was able to use his authority as a medical student to insist that she go. "Well," she said, "If you really think it's necessary, Doctor." Thus, he learned that his responsibility turned out to be neither as all encompassing as he had feared, nor as insignificant as he sometimes imagined.

Nowhere in medicine are the paradoxes more exquisite than in the area of responsibility. At one extreme, students have quite exaggerated notions of their ultimate power. They imagine the practice of medicine as a war constantly being waged on the very cusp of life and death. The training that most students receive in university and charity hospitals, where patients are critically ill, tends to reinforce this harrowing view of responsibility. Usually, students anticipate a time—typically the first day of their internships—when they will have to know everything and be able to do everything, responsible for saving a half a dozen lives a day. Sometimes, faculty reinforce this frightening fantasy.

Professor Ivy, a research microbiologist who didn't care much for teaching medical students anyway, was giving his annual series of lectures on CNS fungi. It was a job his chairman told him he "had to do." The topic of the day was cryptococcal infections.

The lecture was dull and disorganized. Throughout the room, students could be observed yawning, dozing off, or chatting among themselves.

With rising indignation, Professor Ivy interrupted his lecture with this admonition: "You may find this boring now, but wait until you're interns. Some night you're going to be up on the wards and a patient will come in with cryptococcal meningitis. The lab will be closed. *Then* what will you do if you haven't learned how to do an Eaton's India ink stain?!"

As the student's sophistication increases, he begins to realize that responsibility is a concept that goes far beyond TV heroism, however. It is an idea filled with excruciating paradoxes. The student comes to understand that he will be responsible not only for handling the occasional fearsome emergency but also (far more often) for knowing when not to do something. When does a doctor decide not to prolong a child's misery with one more anticancer drug? When does one write the order in a patient's chart, "no heroic measures," or a similar code phrase meaning "allow the patient to die"? When does a doctor decide *not* to take responsibility?

Quinn was a senior student on surgery during an especially hectic admitting night. The hospital was a county hospital, located in a notoriously dangerous section of town. It was Saturday night, the night which the surgery residents cavalierly called "the weekly meeting of the Los Angeles gun and knife club." Two gunshot wounds and a serious stab wound had come up to the floor in rapid succession. In addition, a young woman with a painful breast, presumed to be due to an abscess, had also arrived.

During a hasty 10-minute dinner break, the chief resident had distributed responsibilities. By the time it was decided who would operate on whom, there were no residents left to take care of the young woman with the breast abscess.

"Why don't you do that down in the treatment room, Quinn?" the surgery resident suggested.

Quinn was reluctant. "Well, maybe you'd better help me do my first one."

"Nonsense," the chief resident said. "Here I'll show you!" He then drew a hasty diagram on a napkin with his ballpoint pen showing the presumed location of the abscess and how to make an incision. "Just get to the loculated fluid," he said. "And don't forget to put in a drain."

Two hours later, the resident had to be called out of surgery to come down to the treatment room. Quinn had managed to make a mess of things. The "abscess" had turned out not to be an abscess at all, but a cyst. Quinn's incision had led to a futile groping about for the site of loculated fluid. In addition he had nicked a small artery which he couldn't tie off.

In the end, no mortal harm was done, but the patient had been terribly frightened, subjected to unnecessary pain, and probably had been given a needlessly disfiguring scar.

Quinn was very hard on himself. "How stupid of me!" he ranted to himself. "I should have been responsible enough to say no."

There are many things to say about this disturbing vignette. Quinn himself probably hit on the most important point when he recognized that responsibility also involves knowing one's limitations. Certainly, the system that Quinn found himself in did not make this any easier.

Finally, responsibility is not restricted to knowing what to do (and what not to do). Too often, doctors tend to gravitate toward action. Frequently, the real responsibility that a physician should assume has less to do with action than with his willingness to stand by his patients, making a personal, human commitment to them. Paul did not "do" a great deal for Mrs. Clark in Chapter 1. Yet he did assume a tremendous responsibility, the ethical, human responsibility of staying by her side during her frightening and exquisitely lonely journey toward death.

Paul's instincts about physicianhood were splendid. Yet, he got little help or formal guidance. It is unfortunate that medical school faculty members currently do so little to help students like Paul with their growing sense of responsibility. Not only do we send students hurtling into situations demanding technical expertise that they often do not yet possess—this would be troublesome enough—but, unfortunately, we also fail to help them master responsibility in its broader, human dimension. The doctor's ultimate responsibility lies not in what he can do, but in how humanly committed to people he can be.

Learning a true sense of responsibility is not easy. Students find that they often vacillate between extremes of excessive detachment and excessive involvement. They struggle with the need to be committed to their patients on the one hand while preserving some sense of serenity in their personal lives on the other. At times they feel terribly vulnerable, stripped of their psychological epidermis. At other times, they feel excessively detached, as though they are clanking around in a suit of psychological armor, effective but unwieldy, and purchased at the price of their humanness.

In my view, a major responsibility of ICM courses involves helping students to define responsibility in its most human terms. A further goal should be helping students to integrate growing responsibility in a way that permits the excitement and joy that come from a commitment to patients to flourish. It is unquestionably in his growing ability to be close to patients, and truly responsible for them, that the doctor will discover his greatest meaning. Many current ICM courses represent a heartening step in this direction. More still needs to be done, however, to build on the foundation of the first 2 years. Students in their junior and senior years, interns, and residents are also entitled to help in mastering their responsibility in a way that is enriching rather than traumatic.

ENCOUNTER WITH SEXUALITY

Doctor Snider made a housecall one Saturday morning in response to a request from Miss Pinehurst. Miss Pinehurst stated that she had a bellyache and thought she might need treatment. Doctor Snider, who had come equipped with his medical bag, invited Miss Pinehurst to disrobe. After she had done so, he examined her carefully.

Doctor Snider then decided to give his patient an injection.

At this point things went awry. Miss Pinehurst's mother walked into the room and, with an unmistakable expression of disapproval, told doctor and patient to both get dressed and come to the table for lunch. Doctor Snider and Miss Pinehurst were both 5 years old.

When it comes to the sexual symbolism of medicine, children are far more in touch with it than most adults. If one looks at children playing doctor, in fact, themes of exhibitionism, voyeurism, and sadism (giving a shot is always crucial) emerge regularly.

Where do these feelings later go? Usually they become unconscious. Yet, one must acknowledge that during the long years of medical and residency training, each student will make an odyssey through emotionally intense, often primal experiences—birth, death, pain, madness. They will examine genitals and put their fingers into rectums. It seems hard to imagine that these experiences would not have a great impact. Often, however, the impact is felt primarily at an unconscious level.

Because medical education generally does so little to help students with these experiences, they are left to deal with the eruption of strong unconscious sexual feelings on their own. Generally, one finds three common coping mechanisms:

Humor

Humor is endemic to medicine at all levels of training. Senior skits, for example, are invariably filled with scatological and sexual innuendoes. The anatomy lab is seldom free for long from pranks.

Medical humor has also made its way into the mainstream of contemporary art and literature. The movie *M*A*S*H* (directed by Altman) is a classic example. Especially revealing is the movie's emphasis on sexual voyeurism. A scene in which the soldiers expose a large-breasted, prudish nurse taking a shower to the entire barracks has become something of a classic. Similarly, there is another scene in which one soldier's impotence is cured by staging a mock death, in which he wakes up and believes he is in heaven being seduced by an angel. It is a funny scene. The reason for mentioning it here is that it expresses common concerns that doctors have over their own sexuality. This will be elaborated more under **Changes in Sexuality** below.

Recently, a book entitled *House of God* (Shem) has gained popular notoriety. A vitriolic, powerful depiction of one intern's experience during training, the book has aroused a very mixed response. His black humor describes a journey through hell, one ironically accompanied by many belly laughs. Many medical students and physicians say they have never before read a book that captures so accurately the experience of becoming a doctor. On the other hand, many people who are not physicians have been appalled by the book, very disturbed to think that doctors say and feel such crude, sadistic, and sexual things about their patients. While frequently nonmedical people are frightened and worried by the book, doctors reading it often feel relieved and strangely reassured—reassured most likely because the book helps them realize that they are not alone in their dilemma.

Guilt

For the doctor, guilt takes many forms. Often, the death of a patient can evoke it. The physician may wonder, if only he had studied harder, known more, perhaps things could have been different. Such feelings persist despite evidence to the contrary, even when everyone did all they humanly could.

Students may also feel guilt over their unconscious thoughts and feelings. This is probably what occurred in Dan's dream, at the beginning of the chapter. The cadaver that suddenly lurched forward and pointed an accusing finger at Dan may have stood for Dan's unconscious guilt, reprimanding him for violating the tabooed sanctum of the dead.

We also sometimes experience unconscious responses toward our living patients that may evoke feelings of guilt. It would be a rare student, indeed, who at some point did not become annoyed with a difficult patient. Obnoxious alcoholic patients and psychiatric patients who come into the emergency room after repeated overdoses are classic examples.

Jim was a senior student on emergency medicine when Mildred, a notoriously well known psychiatric patient, came in with her third overdose of Elavil in 6 months. The intern helped Jim initiate the standard measures. An i.v. catheter was inserted and the patient was prepared for gastric lavage. One of the nurses went to get an Ewald tube to insert through the patient's nasopharynx into her stomach.

"Get a big one this time," the intern shouted. "We'll clear out what's left of her nasal turbinates and make it easier for the intern when she comes in next time!"

Jim had laughed, along with the intern and nurse. It was not entirely clear whether Mildred was awake enough to hear, but Jim wasn't sure she hadn't.

More important, he was jolted to realize that he was actually getting some degree of sadistic pleasure from the thought of revenging himself on this patient who seemingly "abused" the medical system, foiling everyone's attempts to help.

Above all, students experience guilt over sexual feelings. Intimate contact with people who are nude—with their genitals, with their bodily secretions—these experiences may put the student into close, often uncomfortable, proximity to his own unconscious sexuality, and this can be guilt provoking.

Changes in Sexual Functioning

The Hollywood image of doctors has it that doctors and nurses are all invariably dashing, physically beautiful people who are constantly going to bed with each other. Again, the film *M*A*S*H* and the subsequent television series are classic examples of this stereotype. Similarly, there is a scene in the Paddy Chayefsky film, *Hospital*, where a philandering intern takes a nurse to bed, while on the other side of the curtain an elderly patient is dying.

In fact, as much as we all might wish to deny it, a great deal of sexual behavior and general flirting do go on as part of ward life, especially during the housestaff years. This is not a popular subject for discussion. Most of us prefer to believe that the image of doctors and nurses on call going to bed with each other is "just Hollywood." In fact, as *House of God* makes clear, it happens repeatedly.

Yet, before we condemn this too harshly, we should try to understand what evokes such behavior. Much of the sexual acting out that goes on between doctors and nurses in hospitals has to do with the intense strain under which they work. Sleepless, beleaguered, overwhelmed by the emotional intensity of what they encounter, they feel frustrated, overwrought, and very vulnerable. The temptation to discharge tension and experience immediate soothing can be very strong. To some, sexual expression seems to be a quick avenue to a bit of stolen comfort, a temporary respite from unbearable tension.

Of course, not every doctor or every nurse partakes in casual sexual liaisons. Often the opposite occurs. Commonly, during certain phases of training, medical students and young doctors find themselves becoming uncharacteristically inhibited. Often, students notice a distressing decline in the frequency of sexual activity. Sometimes such students will try to joke this away, claiming that they are simply "too tired." This can be true, but often the inhibition is related more to an upsurge of unconscious conflict about one's own sexuality, provoked by the clinical work doctors do.

> Donald was a junior on his first OB-GYN rotation. Initially quite anxious about doing pelvics, he soon mastered the procedure and, as far as he could tell, reacted to his daily activities as though they were "old hat." Yet, for a couple of weeks, he seemed to find one excuse or other to avoid going to bed with his wife: he was too tired; he had been on call; there was a journal article he had to read. When his wife confronted him with this, they had attempted to make love and Donald experienced his first episode of impotence.

Experiences of transitory impotence and frigidity are common among students, often alternating with other periods of intense sexuality. Students understandably tend to keep such things to themselves, yet the existence of sexual difficulties is well known, usually expressed in humor. The impotence episode in *M*A*S*H* allowed this subject to be raised, primarily because it was depicted comically. Because transitory alterations in sexuality, due to a student's uncomfortable and often unexpected encounter with his own unconscious, are so common, they should be acknowledged as understandable, human responses to the strain of becoming a doctor.

ACCEPTANCE

In the corny, black and white Hollywood movies of the 30s and 40s, there is often a death scene, and it is often attended by a doctor. Usually there is the obligatory cut to the moment of demise. The doctor shrugs, reveals an expression of sadness, then with resignation pulls the sheet up over the head of the deceased. This signals the end.

If only it were that simple. In fact, all doctors, no matter what their level of experience, will at points anguish over the ultimate caprice of life, its potential for profound unpredictability and unfairness. Even if we could know everything there is to know, there would still be situations that defeat us.

Jeff was a junior medical student on pediatrics when the ambulance arrived with a 9-month-old baby, dead on arrival. The examination was brief, the cause of death quickly revealed. Long bone x-rays showed multiple old fractures, and the skull x-ray, one massive new one. The child had been battered to death.

Enraged, furious, and overwhelmed by a feeling of helplessness, Jeff stormed out of the examining room where the dead child lay into the hall to confront its mother. There he saw a slender, sobbing, 16-year-old girl, still a child herself, weeping inconsolably in the corner.

No longer knowing whom to hate, whom to blame, Jeff ran into a room where he would be undiscovered and wept.

Life plays tricks. Car wrecks kill good people as well as bad people. Cancer strikes the brave and noble as well as the mediocre and ignominious. If there is a sense to be discerned in life's patterns, it will be found in religion and philosophy, not in medicine. Yet medicine exposes us constantly to all of life's cruelest, most unexpected tricks. Not surprisingly, it is often the most sensitive student who feels the pain of this the most.

The ultimate integration of these realities can bring to a physician what we crudely call "wisdom." To the sensitive student, it can also bring periods of anguish, rage, vulnerability, and pain. Certainly, Paul felt all of these when Mrs. Clark died. Yet, after he cried, he experienced something else—a sense of acceptance that did not feel the same as defeat. It was this acceptance that led him to feel he was becoming a doctor.

Ultimately, it is through standing with our patients, sharing with them in the puzzling and sometimes lethal mystery of their illness, that we achieve our highest purpose as doctors. This is expressed most eloquently by Lorin L. Stephens, an orthopaedist and clinical professor at the University of Southern California School of Medicine who, until his death in 1974, was a beloved and admired inspiration to countless students and young doctors:

There are those who will tell you that being a physician is a curse, a life of endless and ambiguous work, where at best we are consumed in a holding action—and all that, without experiencing appropriate appreciation of our sacrifice.

I do not feel that way. Being a physician I consider the highest privilege I can imagine. Along with the joys from my family, my life as a physician has provided me with moments of epiphany, transcendental moments of lucidity . . . To be a physician—to be permitted to be invited by another human being into his life in the circumstances of that crucible which is illness—to be a trusted participant in the highest of dramas—for these privileges I am grateful beyond my ability to express . . .

References

Altman, R. (Dir.): *M*A*S*H*, 20th Century Fox, 1970.

Cousins, N.: The doctor as artist and philosopher (Editorial). *Saturday Review*, July 22, 1978, p. 56.

Hiller, A. (Dir.): *Hospital*, script by Paddy Chayefsky, United Artists, 1971.

Keniston, K.: The medical student. *Yale J. Biol. Med. 39:*6, 1967.

Knight, J. A.: *Medical Student. Doctor in the Making*, Meredith Corp., Appleton-Century-Crofts, New York, 1973.

Lewin, B. D.: Counter-transference in the technique of medical practice. *Psychosom. Med. 8:* 195, 1946.

Sexton, Anne: *The Awful Rowing Toward God*, Houghton Mifflin Co., Boston, 1975.

Sheehy, G.: *Passages: Predictable Crises of Adult Life*, E.P. Dutton & Co., New York, 1976.

Shem, S.: *The House of God*, Richard Merek Publishers, New York, 1978.

Werner, E. R., and Korsch, B. M.: The vulnerability of the medical student: Posthumous presentation of L.L. Stephens' ideas. *Pediatrics 57:*321, 1976.

chapter 3

BECOMING A PATIENT

LONELINESS

No sky at all,
No earth at all—and still
the snowflakes fall . . .
Masaoka Shiki

In the spring of my senior year of medical school, I became ill. For a time I was quite sick, though at first I did not realize it and later would not admit it. The illness, in fact, had some potential for being fatal.

In this chapter, I discuss my own experience with this illness. To do so directly and undefensively is not easy. As I approach the task, I feel more anxiety than I anticipated; it is surprisingly painful to recall the events and feelings I thought I had mastered and put permanently behind me. To remember is to acknowledge that my future was once in jeopardy. To reawaken the vulnerability I felt then is to admit that I could become vulnerable again—at any time—and this frightens me.

Though I am a physician—perhaps because I am a physician—I still try to deny my own human frailty as much as possible. I am remembering now as I write that, during the years following that serious incident, when I occasionally had a gastrointestinal virus, the question always passed through my mind: "Is it happening again?" As soon as I was better, this thought was just as quickly forgotten. I still try to minimize the impact that being sick has had on me.

There is little precedent in medical literature for using one's self as a case history. This may be due in part to understandable apprehensions about self-disclosure. I certainly have some concerns about this. To disclose my physical and psychological vulnerabilities of that time causes me to feel somehow shameful, a feeling that persists despite its illogic. Also, my illness involved

45

the gastrointestinal tract, provoking special concerns over revealing things that are "dirty" and therefore embarrassing.

However, a more important reason for the paucity of personal statements in the literature probably stems from our notions of science and objectivity. On the surface of it, to talk about the emotions one felt at the height of a painful and frightening illness seems hopelessly unobjective. But unobjective may not mean inaccurate. It is arguable that, in trying to understand something as personal and ultimately singular as the experience of being ill, there may be some value in seeing things through the patient's eyes, as only the patient can.

Sometimes only a doctor can best understand another doctor. It may also be that, from certain perspectives, only a patient can truly understand another patient. I say this, having spent considerable effort as a physician trying to understand patients, from a doctor's point of view. Having been on both sides, I have developed a strong conviction that doctors who are practicing effectively cannot, and should not, become so welded to their patients psychologically that they feel no difference between their patients' pain and their own. In order to help people who are sick, we must know what it is like to be in their shoes but, at the same time, also know very well that we are *not* in their shoes. A 25-year-old intern treating a 25-year-old man with leukemia should be able to empathize with what it feels like to be that age and very possibly dying; yet, it is also essential that the intern know that he is not dying himself.

What I am describing is almost a spatial relationship between the doctor and his patients. Where do we stand? Do we hover far away, viewing them from the safe distance of objectivity and detachment, scrutinizing them through the wrong end of a telescope, and restricting our involvement to handling diseased tissues and managing disturbed serum levels? Or, at the other extreme, do we merge with our patients? With each patient's pain, do we ache unbearably? Are we consigned to die a thousand deaths if we allow ourselves to get close? Clearly, the answer is that we must learn to dwell somewhere between these extremes. Yet, I think, to many students and young doctors, this advice sounds like a hollow cliché. In truth, students experience almost incessant swings between overidentification and excessive detachment in their work with patients. Even at later points in our professional development, none of us is immune from these swings. I do believe, however, that with time and support from colleagues, we can begin to achieve a stance that permits us to feel with our patients yet not become one with them. This stance has been described variously as the difference between empathy and sympathy, between understanding and identification—the achievement of "detached concern." However we name it, achieving this stance is one of the most difficult tasks we must master as physicians; yet, achieving such a balance is essential for our own personal peace and for the effective care of our patients. Even the most empathic physician will, therefore, set necessary limits to the amount of pain he permits himself to feel in his care of the sick. Unless he becomes sick himself. In that situation, I truly believe that the physician cannot be a doctor to himself, regardless of how much he knows about disease. Instead, he becomes the patient.

The loneliness of being sick is almost inexpressible. The doctor's power to reach through that loneliness and be with his patient for a while is one of his most mysterious, potent, and potentially curative tools. Yet, finally, he leaves and the patient is alone. He would not really want the doctor to stay. If he did, he could not provide effective care. There can be no doubt that illness means separation of a most profound and fundamental kind.

In the film *Black Orpheus*, there is a powerful scene in which Orpheus finds himself lost in a decaying office building in downtown Rio de Janeiro. It is late at night. He is alone in the building. All the employees have gone. He is searching in vain for Eurydice. In the fading light, he searches among endless shelves, row upon row of rotting, forgotten archives. He is looking for her in the Bureau of Statistics. Everywhere, moldering on the shelves in silence, are the forgotten slips of paper that recorded a life, marked down a death. The task is futile.

Meanwhile, somewhere in the streets of Rio, caught up in the mad swirl of Mardi Gras, Eurydice is also lost. Death is lurking in the shadows with an ironic smile on his face, doggedly tracking her down. Though she is engulfed by revelers, she too is utterly alone. In terror, she vainly cries out for her beloved Orpheus.

This scene appears to me a wrenching symbol of our own isolation from those we love during our final, inevitable, and losing struggle against death.

One final image: back in the deserted office building, Orpheus encounters another living figure. It is a hobbled, aging janitor, pushing scraps of paper from one meaningless location in the building to another. He listens sympathetically to Orpheus' plight. Yet both are obviously helpless. The janitor ruefully gestures about him, musing at the meaninglessness of all the statistics, all the fading pages of forgotten print. Then, he is gone.

I certainly do not wish to suggest that as physicians we are as lost and hopelessly bewildered as Orpheus. Yet I do think we share with him some limitations. We too sometimes feel like Orpheus, like the janitor, solitary figures moving scraps of paper against the backdrop of mortality itself. And our patients, caught in the swirling activity of a busy hospital ward, may also feel something of Eurydice's loneliness and terror.

If we are to be truly compassionate toward our patients, we must understand that, though we can share with them for a time, in the end, our patients face their suffering, their illness, and sometimes their death alone.

*   *   *   *

My story begins so subtly that I cannot tell you the precise point when I first became ill. It was toward the end of May, or the first part of June, 1972. I had recently taken Part II of the National Board Exams and was a senior on Pediatrics—my last rotation before graduation.

It was a joyous time in my life. I was graduating from medical school. I had been accepted into the residency training program of my choice. I was rotating on Peds with some of my good friends, feeling perhaps a little sad at our upcoming separation but mostly very happy to be experiencing a sense of mastery and to be sharing this with people I cared about. Perhaps most exciting was my upcoming graduation address, for which my class had selected me. I naturally felt complimented by their choice, but beyond that, I saw a real opportunity to express for all of us what going to medical school had meant. I was also a bit nervous, anticipating the writing I had yet to do and the prospect of speaking before such a large gathering. In fact, it was to this nervousness that I attributed the initial symptoms of my illness.

The first symptoms I recall specifically occurred in the morning, during bedside rounds. I remember the occasion, though not the exact day, because we were rounding, as we always did, near the bedside of a little 11-year-old boy named Greg. Greg was dying of leukemia.

Here was a distressing situation. Greg was not actually a patient on our service. Nor was he a patient on anyone's service up where we were. We were working on Infectious Disease, and our ward had the only effective isolation units. As a consequence of his chemotherapy, Greg had experienced a marked leukopenia and increased susceptibility to infection. It had therefore been decided to "house" him on our unit, in isolation.

The isolation bed was actually a glassed-in enclosure that jutted out into the ward like a transparent parapet. He could see out, though he never looked at us, and we could see in. He had his own TV, which was always on, tuned to an endless stream of detergent commercials and daytime quiz shows. Greg never watched. He had many soft, plush stuffed animals on his bed.

I believe the enclosure had been designed with the most humane of intentions. Most probably the architect felt this would be a design that would leave the patient feeling less cutoff from the parade of humanity beyond the foot of his bed. In actuality, it was a surreal prison. I never saw anyone in there with him except hospital personnel. Perhaps it was the time of day we saw him, but I suspect his vigil was a lonely one.

The little boy was terribly depressed. Morning after morning, I would watch him lying there, staring out into space, the ice blue reflection of the unwatched TV set flickering on his face. I longed to go in, yet was terrified to do so. I was able to say to myself, "He's not my patient." What disturbed me most was the grave, cruelly inappropriate expression of maturity in his eyes. One look and you could tell—this child knew he was going to die.

When we would round on other patients near Greg, I would always find my attention drifting until I was once again transfixed on this ashen-faced little boy who never seemed to move or smile. The only time I saw him cry was when an intern had to do a cut-down on him to restart his i.v. He would die before my rotation ended.

I was staring in at Greg one morning, as I always did, when I felt a twinge of pain deep in my abdomen. It was a cramping sensation. Too much coffee, I thought to myself, or something. I also noticed a burning, itching sensation that felt like it was originating deep in my rectum. The cramping was intense. Surprisingly so. For a few minutes I tried to ignore it. I leaned against the railing of a nearby bed, hunching over a bit, and tried to pay attention to rounds. For some reason, I felt embarrassed. Above all, I didn't want anyone to know I was in distress. After several minutes, however, I had to excuse myself and hurried to the bathroom.

After I had moved my bowels, it seemed slightly strange to me that the cramping did not go away. For the next half-hour or so I continued to experience pain. After about an hour, however, the symptoms abated and I forgot all about them for the remainder of the day.

In the ensuing days, however, the same symptoms were to recur with maddening regularity. I had never had any such change in bowel habits before, yet I rationalized everything as being due to anxiety about my upcoming talk.

The symptoms gradually got worse. I could almost set my clock by their onset each day. Every morning between 9:00 and 9:30, I would experience deep, intense cramping pain in my lower abdomen. This would be accompanied by a strong sensation of burning and itching in my rectum. However, several other changes had also begun to occur. Now, every morning I would experience strong urges to evacuate my bowels; but there would be no bowel movement. Instead, there would be water and mucous occasionally tinged with blood. The burning was getting worse, and the cramps were persisting longer. Still, everything would clear up by about noon, and I would spend the rest of the day symptom-free.

About a week and a half after the appearance of my first symptoms, my wife and I went out to dinner with friends. I recall the occasion vividly; this was the night that my denial began to break down.

It was a rare clear night in Los Angeles. We could see all the way to the San Gabriel Mountains from the medical school and all of my friends were in a good mood. The evening was balmy and the air filled with jasmine. By now, however, my cramping was persisting through the entire day, and I was in too much discomfort to enjoy a splendid sunset.

I had also begun to lose weight and at times would experience dizziness when I exerted myself. Normal bowel movements had ceased. Instead, I would frequently pass copious amounts of fluid and mucuous. The traces of blood were now consistently present.

I had described these symptoms that night—a bit ashamedly—to my friend and classmate, John. To my relief, John had encouraged me not to worry.

"Why don't you just try to forget about it this evening," he exhorted. "Have a good time."

I also got the distinct feeling that John did not want to believe that I could really be sick.

We went to a popular restaurant, a noisy place with sawdust and peanut shells on the floor, crowds, loud conversation, and lots of beer. I tried to smile and act involved in the conversation; but, as was becoming increasingly true then, my mind was elsewhere. I was absorbed by my illness, especially by the continuous experience of pain. During soup, I excused myself and hurried to the bathroom.

I knew then that I was sick. I sat for a long time in one of the bathroom stalls, doubled over, pressing my head against my knees, weeping, praying for the pain to stop. It went on and on. Outside the booth, I could hear the door slamming. I listened to people come and go, friends chatting, people washing up before dinner, the sound of healthy people having a good time. Through the stall, I could glimpse pairs of shoes, bottoms of trousers. With tears in my eyes, I fought back hard against a growing panic.

I felt trapped, in jeopardy, embarrassed, furious, and envious—all at the same time. Above all, I felt isolated, locked in not by a latch but by my pain. Beyond the door were "normal" people, people free of illness and pain, people I could not join.

After what must have been a quarter of an hour, John came in and asked if anything was wrong.

"No," I lied. "I'm OK. Just a bit of cramping."

I urged him to return to the table and reassure my wife and friends that I was OK—just had "a bug" or something—and would rejoin them soon.

I was unable to return to dinner that night, however, and felt compelled instead to go out to the car we had come in and lie down. There, at least, I could be alone, free of the pressure to maintain a pretense. I longed for darkness, cool, and quiet. This reaction became typical of my feelings as my illness got worse. A great deal of the time I just wanted to be left alone. I preferred things as quiet and unstimulating as possible. I could only find energy to concentrate on reducing my pain.

Almost simultaneously, however, I would have an opposite reaction, so much so that I found my relationship to my friends, and even my wife, becoming increasingly fraught with paradoxes. I became increasingly demanding and dependent, especially on my wife. I would make frequent, righteous demands. For example, lying in the car that night, outside the restaurant doubled up in pain, I was furious: furious at my wife for not leaving the table and joining me in my vigil, and furious at my friend, John, for taking me at my word when I had said, "Go ahead and enjoy yourselves, don't mind me." I was furious that everyone had not rushed to my side. Yet had they, I would have felt claustrophobic and regarded their concern as an intrusion.

After what seemed like an eternity that evening, my friends did return. Later, when we arrived home, I told my wife, "I think I'm sick. Maybe we'd better call a doctor."

But I did not call a doctor. I reasoned that my complaints were not important enough to warrant a call at night. Also, as is so typical of medical students and physicians, I actually had no doctor. Most of the minor physical complaints that had bothered me during medical school I had treated by grabbing a resident and getting some antibiotics or by just ignoring them until they went away.

The following morning, I finally did call an internist. He was a clinical professor at my medical school and had done a routine physical on me when I was a freshman. I hadn't consulted him in 4 years, but he came closest to being my doctor.

It was a Saturday, and I initially got his answering service. He returned my call about an hour later. I could tell on the phone that he was trying to remember me, though I don't know if he ever really succeeded. I described my symptoms. Although I depicted them accurately, I found myself playing down my concern, speaking in a tone that conveyed levity. I said I was "probably being psychosomatic." That term was big in my vocabulary in those days. Whenever my wife would feel sick, I would accuse her of "being psychosomatic." Looking back on it, I think that my constant exposure as a medical student to illness and death had left me inwardly terrified. When my wife or I experienced a physical symptom of illness I would try to reduce my fear by denying the possibility that anything could really be wrong—it must just be "psychosomatic."

After I described my symptoms, Dr. Burgess was silent for a moment. Then, following what seemed some indecision on his part, he suggested that I take Donnagel with paragoric and call him during the week if "things don't clear by then."

Of course, they didn't. Over the weekend, I became increasingly ill and reacted by becoming increasingly obstinate and irrascible. My symptoms had begun to alarm my wife. She had somewhat timidly suggested, "Maybe you'd better call him back, or go to the emergency room." I, in turn, had lashed out at her for being "too anxious." Yet, in the next breath, I found myself demanding constant attention from her, in the form of bringing me broth, tea, and my doses of medicine (which, incidentally, did no good).

Rather than seek medical attention, I decided to "study" my problem. In between trips to the john, I got out my Harrison's *Textbook of Medicine* and my Cecil and Loeb, and I took copious notes.

Gradually, I developed my own differential diagnosis. Here are what the notes looked like:

1. infectious diarrhea: a strong rule-out. Perhaps most likely. Atypical for amoebiasis—possibly bacterial. Exposure to one of my patients possible. Get stool culture. Stools for O & P.
2. functional diarrhea: less likely, but always a R/O. Certainly several stresses recently. Could be psychosomatic. Hx of other episode relative to stress? Sm. caliber stools?
3. diverticulitis: disease of elderly. Less severe pain. Otherwise—Sx fit.
4. ulcerative colitis: a remote R/O. Hx not typical. Abdominal cramping rarely that severe c̄ C.U.C.

On Monday I was unable to go to school. That day an event occurred that I will always remember as one of the most terrifying of my life. On about my fifth trip of the morning to the bathroom, I stood up and suddenly felt extremely dizzy. The room began to spin and, as I tried to grab onto something, I fell to the floor and passed out. When I tried to get up, it started to happen again. I finally had to crawl on my hands and knees to get back to my bed. I realized, to my horror, that the days of fluid loss, exhaustion, and poor hydration had weakened me. It occurred to me that I might even be in electrolyte imbalance. For the first time, I took my temperature; it was mildly elevated, about 99.6°. I knew then that I had to get help.

I got the name of a gastroenterologist, Dr. Axelrod, from one of my professors. I called him immediately. Initially, I was unable to get past his receptionist, who protected him zealously from patients like me. She offered me an appointment in 3 weeks. By this time, however, I had some grasp of my situation and insisted, with some hint of a threat, that I speak to the doctor directly. I invoked what little authority I had as a medical student.

Finally, I did get to speak with the doctor, and he gave me an appointment for later that afternoon. I still often wonder what would have happened to someone in my predicament who had been less assertive and more easily backed down by bureaucratic officiousness.

Much of the rest of that day is now a blur in my memory. What I do recall most distinctly are the sigmoidoscopy and the talk I had in Dr. Axelrod's office afterwards. I had always dreaded the prospect of sigmoidoscopy, and, in fact, the examination was excruciating despite the doctor's gentleness and technical finesse. During it, I briefly passed out again.

Afterwards Dr. Axelrod asked me into his office, a richly panelled, leather-upholstered affair befitting his prominence. I asked him what he thought. With a look of unmistakable gravity and compassion, he told me, "You have chronic ulcerative colitis."

During the dialogue that followed, I was completely devoid of any conscious feeling. With great detachment, I carefully posed a number of succinct questions. It was as though I were consulting on some patient other than myself.

"How bad does it appear?" I asked.

"Fairly severe," he said.

"Do I have to go into the hospital?"

"No—you need strict bed rest and steroids. I want to keep a close eye on you, but I don't think you need to go into the hospital yet."

"Yet?"

"We'll have to watch you carefully."

I then asked two questions related to prognosis.

"What is the likelihood of an eventual operation?"

"Thirty to fifty percent. But remember these are just statistics."

"Am I at greater risk for colonic cancer?"

"Yes."

"Will this shorten my lifetime?"

"It may, yes."

Interestingly, there was one question I did not ask. I think it was simply too terrifying to consider. I did not inquire whether I might become too sick to continue training, too sick to be a doctor.

In the ensuing weeks, I never panicked, never experienced anxiety that I was aware of. I never once cried. To the contrary, I experienced great relief. For one thing, I had been overwhelmingly relieved that I did not have to enter the hospital. Also, I had begun a regimen of Azulfidine and steroids. Within several days, I was experiencing great symptomatic relief. Finally, to be in less pain was incredibly liberating. In contrast to my agony of the week before, I was now in a state of mild euphoria, possibly enhanced by the steroids.

As for the grim prognostications, I began to think that perhaps Dr. Axelrod had been too hasty. The stool cultures still weren't back. It might still be infectious. Even if it were ulcerative colitis, I had read in several sources that, in rare cases, the disease spontaneously remits and does not pursue a chronic course. I was sure that mine was such a case.

Still, in that first week after being diagnosed, I had two very vivid dreams.

In the first dream, it is fall. I am very happy, walking through a stand of woods. Dry leaves crunch and crackle with my footsteps. The weather is crisp and the sky a deep azure blue. There is that delicious burning leave smell of autumn air. I am suddenly, inexplicably, at the bottom of a deep well. The sides are rough-hewn and composed of dark gray granite. At the rim I can see a patch of sky—white cumulus clouds drift by. Faces appear. They seem concerned, but do not stay. I shout up at them, asking them to bring help, but they cannot hear me. My wife appears. She asks me how long I have to stay down there and appears to be worried. Then, she shouts down to me, "I see you. I know you're in trouble, David. I'm coming!" She begins to climb over the rim. In sudden terror, I shout to her, "Turn back, danger! Don't come down here! The dream ends.

In the second dream, I am swimming laps in a pool. I am feeling strong and exultant. I guide myself by means of a black line painted onto the tiles along the bottom of the pool. Gradually, the line drops off into deeper water. Everything suddenly darkens. To my horror, I am suddenly lost in deep, dark, murky water. In the distance, I spot a shark. It swims slowly, almost luxuriously, in my direction. I grope desperately for the surface, but I am fathoms below it and suddenly trapped in a labyrinth of seaweed.

The only other time that my denial failed me during that period was one afternoon when my wife knocked over our typewriter. I had been on bed rest and was still quite weak. Because I had trouble sitting up and typing, my wife had graciously agreed to type large parts of my speech as I managed to scribble it down on paper. We were living in a small rented house at the time, filled with the usual rickety mixture of Goodwill hand-me-downs, boards and bricks, and junky "antiques." My wife had placed our Smith-Corona portable on the top of one such antique, a narrow, flimsy pedestal table. This apparatus, in turn, was poised at the edge of the bed so she could type while keeping me company. The electric cord stretched precariously across the length of the floor.

During my illness and especially in my beginning convalescence, I had become extremely self-indulgent. My egocentricity showed itself everywhere, but I did not especially question it or even seem particularly aware of it. In fact, my wife's typing draft after redraft of my speech, day after day, represented a lot of work for her, in addition, she now had to cook all the meals, keep track of my medications, and help administer steroid enemas to me—all on top of working fulltime. I think, as well, that she was using far less denial than I was then, though we never discussed it. I am sure, in fact, that I was quite insensitive to her own experience of loneliness, depression, and fear. At the time, all that she was doing for me simply seemed my due.

One might, I suppose, just chalk this up to male chauvinism. I certainly practiced my share. But I think it would be more accurate to say that I had regressed. I had ceased to relate to my wife as an equal and instead regarded her with the implicit conviction that I was her child and she was my mother. I found this relationship very reassuring. Doubtless, it also rendered me a demanding, whiny, self-centered brat for large stretches of time with little capacity to reciprocate as an adult to my spouse, who was experiencing pain and needs of her own as a result of my illness.

On one especially hectic day, she was in a rush and tripped on the typewriter cord, toppling the table and smashing the typewriter onto the floor with a loud clatter.

I leapt from the bed and ran to its rescue. Cradling it in my arms as though it were a sick child, I lamented its injuries. The carriage had been badly bent. Bursting into tears, I wept angrily and accused her of "ruining everything." Like a 3-year-old having a tantrum, I moaned that now I'd "never be able to do my speech."

In her turn, my exhausted wife burst into tears herself, hurtled my notepad at me, and shouted "Write your own damned speech." She left the house and went on a long walk.

As I reflect on this now, I am embarrassed to remember a time when I was so regressed, infantile, and narcissistic. Yet, I had been denying huge anxieties, on many levels, by fixating on my upcoming speech. Like the drunk who can focus only on getting his key into the keyhole while the world is spinning around him, I seemed to be keeping my sights riveted exclusively to my upcoming speech. The typewriter crashing down symbolized reality; it symbolized the loss of my defenses; ultimately I believe it symbolized the failure of my own body. Unable as I was then to accept the deeper terror that this implied, I chose instead to blame it on my wife as though there might be some comfort in laying blame for my predicament.

In the end, the speech went well. I was still on steroids. In addition, I was taking codeine for diarrhea and pain. Together, I think they left me feeling slightly out of it a good deal of the time. Still, I was able to "pull it off." This had become the consuming goal: to pull things off, to be able to stand on my own feet, to hide my infirmity. Interestingly, the speech itself had a lot to do with how doctors and students often need to deny things. Yet, if someone had suggested that I was talking about myself, I would have looked at him as though he had just landed from Mars.

I recall a snapshot that was taken that day. I am standing proudly dressed up in my cap and gown, but thin, haggard, and conspicuously pale. I had absolutely no awareness of how bad I looked then. The photo still shocks me.

* * * *

The following days and weeks form something of a blur in my memory. My wife and I soon packed and left for Colorado where I was to begin residency training. It was a time of tremendous anticipation and excitement. I recall finding great splendor and beauty in the vast, arid deserts of Nevada and Utah, which we crossed on our car trip to Denver. I had plenty of time to enjoy these vistas, incidentally, for I was still too weak to drive. In addition, I had become accustomed to hanging those plastic bags full of steroid enema every night from the corners of nondescript motel paintings in every Holiday Inn from L.A. to Trinidad, Colorado. I seemed to be adjusting.

Upon arriving in Denver, one of the first orders of business was to make an appointment with a local gastroenterologist who would follow my illness. I had been referred by Dr. Axelrod to a friend of his in Denver; he in turn referred me to a young assistant professor in the Department of Medicine at the University of Colorado, Dr. Singleman. I introduced myself to him quite simply. "I'm David Reiser. I have ulcerative colitis."

As part of his evaluation, he again performed the dreaded sigmoidoscopy. This time, I was in less pain and was much less regressed psychologically. My reactions to the procedure were, therefore, different, though still striking. I was less concerned about the pain this time than I was about my dignity. Dr. Singleman was assisted by an attractive nurse in her mid-20s. While I still feared the pain of the procedure, what I remember most vividly is my embarrassment at being subjected to it in front of a pretty young woman.

Dr. Singleman, I recall, was somewhat perplexed. He told me that the sigmoidoscopic findings "could be ulcerative colitis, but don't look like what I've usually seen." He took a biopsy specimen. For the first time since my illness had begun, I was asked for a drug history.

Was I taking any medications?

At first I answered, no. Then, as he pressed me, I did recall a seemingly trivial episode, long since forgotten. Approximately 3 weeks before the onset of my earliest symptoms, I had been troubled by a minor dermatologic cyst. In my typical fashion, I had nabbed a dermatology resident in the hallway who, in turn, handed me a 10-day supply of a relatively new antibiotic he had gotten from a detail man. The drug was Cleocin. I had taken it for 10 days, and the cyst had cleared. At least 2 weeks passed between the last dose of the drug and the onset of my first symptoms. I had therefore never linked the two in my mind. Still, to Dr. Singleman, this seemed significant.

At that time, data on Cleocin were relatively scanty and new. Since then, Cleocin has become well recognized for this serious, occasionally fatal, side-effect. I will always be very thankful to Dr. Singleman, not only for his decent treatment of me, but also for his knowledge, intuition, and skepticisim.

*   *   *   *

It turned out that I did not have ulcerative colitis, for which I thank God. At least, there has been no recurrence of any symptoms since the original episode in 1972.

So, the story has a happy ending.

I recall a conversation with my parents shortly after the illness had been rediagnosed.

My mother had exclaimed, "We're so relieved!" She went on to say that both she and my father had worried about whether such an illness would affect my ability to practice consistently as a physician. My mother, a nurse, may have been worrying too much. Yet, I do remember that conversation with a chill. Until I was safe, I had never allowed myself to consider the very real possibility that my disease might not only deprive me of my life and large sections of my bowel, but also of my ability to function as a physician.

I would like to close this chapter with two thoughts.

First, for many years, I have used the experience of my own illness to teach my students. In particular, I have used it to underscore the importance of diagnostic caution and thorough history-taking. It is a classic example of how patients in general, and doctors in particular, resist getting appropriate medical care. Finally, I have always felt that this story underscores the hazards of facile psychologizing about illness.

As one might imagine, during the period when I thought I had ulcerative colitis, I did a great deal of reading in various texts and became something of an expert on the syndrome. I learned, among other things, that ulcerative colitis is considered a "psychosomatic illness." I recall all too well a description in one well known textbook of the so-called "ulcerative colitis personality." The ulcerative colitis personality was described by this author as immature looking, unable to form close relationships, a passive-aggressive individual who is riddled by anger, resentment, and inhibitions and who cannot express his needs directly; instead he is covert, sneaky, and passive. This is a patient, the author said, who will smile when you come into the room and then spit in your face.

At the time, I was stung by this description. For one thing, I felt terribly misunderstood. The description didn't fit me; yet, since I had the disease, it must be true about me. I even tried to rethink myself, to reformulate my self-concept to fit a textbook description. After all, if this was the opinion of a major textbook in the field, it must be true, and I must learn to accept it. But, it never did fit. Beyond this, even if the description had been accurate, it would not have hurt any less. The words were cruel and laden with pious value judgments. They did nothing to help. I envisioned a lifetime of contact with physicians who would regard me as passive-aggressive. Somehow, above all, the notion of psychosomatic seemed to imply that I was (in some mysterious way) guilty of a psychological "original sin." It is hard to describe the shame and isolation that a patient feels when he reads something like that.

What I am saying is in no sense intended to denigrate the psychological underpinnings of many diseases. It is my own belief that many illnesses, mental and physical alike, have antecedents in psychological stress, among other important factors. Yet, I must say that I experienced the simplistic psychologizing of several textbooks as hurtful and unempathic—a cheap shot. It makes me wonder how many other patients, with so-called "classic" psychosomatic disorders, have been subjected to such prejudice.

I have made this point to many of my students. Yet, if I am to be completely honest, I must close by also making a second point. It occurs to me now, from the safety of considerable retrospection, that a number of things *were* going on in my life at that time. I was graduating from medical school. I was about to give a speech that was very important to me. I was beginning residency training. While it is true that I took a drug that has since been shown to be toxic, I wonder whether other psychological factors *didn't* enter in. Would I have contracted the same illness had I not been anxious about many important events at the time? I cannot answer this question, but I think it reasonable to raise it. I wonder—and I know I will never test this hypothesis—if I took Cleocin again, under very different circumstances, would my bowel react to it in the same way? I don't think anyone knows the answer. I do know that, for the brief period of time when I thought I had this disease, I believe my reactions were in many ways classical; they included denial, regression, self-centeredness, and a need to maintain control. Above all, I experienced deep loneliness.

I cannot make any claim to speak for other patients; I can only say what my becoming ill meant to me. Several things stand out in my mind: the anguish of chronic pain (it can make anyone wish he were dead); the helplessness and loss of control; the overwhelming self-centeredness; the equally overwhelming dependence– on other people, on drugs, on doctors, on sigmoidoscopes—and, above all, the isolation, the knowledge that you alone will live or die from what you've got. Others may come close and sympathize. A physician, with his knowledge and empathy, can offer a special kind of optimism and hope. Yet, even a doctor has his limits. For me, the most towering, most impenetrable, most compelling significance of illness lies in the knowledge that ultimately each of us must live his life and face his death, alone. For a short time, I believe I knew what it was like to be Greg, to be 11 and dying; for a mercifully brief period, I understood what it means to be on the other side of that ineffable glass window that separates the well from the sick and the living from the dying.

References

Camus, M. (Dir.): *Black Orpheus*, Lopert Films release, 1959.

Henderson, H. G.: *An Introduction to Haiku*, Doubleday Anchor Books, New York, 1958.

Lief, H. I., and Fox, R. C.: Training for "Detached Concern" in medical students. In *The Psychological Basis of Medical Practice*, edited by Harold I. Lief, Victor L. Lief, and Nina R. Lief, Hoeber Medical Division, Harper and Row, New York, 1963.

chapter 4

REACTIONS TO ILLNESS

ILLNESS AS DEVELOPMENT

If one examines pre-Renaissance paintings of children closely, something striking becomes apparent: they are not paintings of children at all. Instead, one sees miniature adults, scaled down in size but lacking the proportions of children. The roundness of a child's face, the immaturity of the nose are not well captured. One sees the face of an adult.

What these paintings fail to reflect is a concept of development. Just as medieval artists could not represent depth of field in their paintings until they had a concept of perspective, they also could not paint children without an awareness of development.

A concept of development is also integral to our understanding of patients. For example, the development of the speciality of pediatrics grew out of a recognition that children differ from adults—anatomically, physiologically, in their patterns of susceptibility to disease, and in their response to treatment.

We now know a great deal more about the development of children; but, until very recently, we neglected to recognize continuing development in the adult and typically halted our analysis at late childhood or adolescence. Erik Erikson advanced knowledge in this area considerably when, in 1950, he proposed that developmental stages continue to unfold throughout one's adult life and into old age. Since then, Vaillant, Levenson, and others have expanded our knowledge of development in the adult.

I would like to propose that illness itself can be viewed from the perspective of development. Perhaps the best known example of this kind of perspective is contained in the work of Elisabeth Kübler-Ross, whose conception of the stages of dying is now widely and deservedly esteemed. When I speak here of a developmental perspective, I am obviously not referring to psychosexual stages or even to broadly defined phases of adulthood. Rather, I am referring

59

to the fact that, during the course of illness, a patient is subjected to major internal and external changes which cause a disruption in the way the patient previously viewed himself and the world. This disruption, in turn, demands that the patient adapt, either by growing psychologically and developing a new perspective or by retreating and pulling away from life. That this process can be excruciatingly painful is clear. Yet, there is also potential for maturation, increased wisdom, and personal growth.

It is in this broader sense that I use the term development when I speak of patients' reactions to illness. One fruitful way of looking at patients' responses to illness—and not just to fatal illness—is as a crisis in development. In the course of becoming ill, the patient undergoes an evolution. The way in which he adapts has great implications for his clinical management and for his future quality of life. We do not often change willingly or without struggle. Illness forces upon an individual the absolute necessity of change. Some of us will inevitably adapt better than others. The question is, can the physician have a positive role in this process? Can he, beyond his knowledge of his patient's disease, offer a special kind of relationship that will help his patient adapt to illness as positively as possible?

Cassell has proposed that four phenomena are central to the experience of being ill: loss of connection, loss of a sense of omnipotence, the failure of reason, and loss of control. In a very sensitive way, he makes it clear that the pain and suffering of the ill person are, at heart, *human* experiences, not simply instances of psychopathology. To Cassell's categories I would add several others, including ambivalence about knowing, turning inward, rebellion, and, especially, shattering of identity. These experiences, too, are first and foremost human reactions to illness, not evidence of further sickness in our patients.

In the following pages, I will discuss a number of reactions that patients commonly have to illness from the perspective of development. Illness is not static. It is a highly dynamic process that evolves over time, with stages through which a patient will typically progress; reactions to illness are best understood from such a perspective.

It is necessary at this point to define development more precisely, since the term is used in different ways. The most classical definition is derived from embryology. It states, basically, that development proceeds in a fixed, biologically innate sequence and at a genetically determined rate. Progressively, in a stepwise fashion, an organism develops from a stage of minimal anatomical and functional differentiation to a stage of maximal anatomical and functional complexity.

Over time, this definition has gradually been broadened to encompass concepts of psychological development, especially in children. An example is the concept of the development of independence: between the ages of approximately 1 and 3, a child experiences rapid growth and development of his neuromusculature. This growth, which is genetically determined and biologically innate, results in increased strength, motility, and coordination; in short, the child begins to walk. From this, psychological developments ensue. The child begins to separate more from his mother, at first literally, being able to walk farther and farther from her, and later, symbolically.

Thus, from an innate biological thrust, psychological growth has naturally followed. Other similar examples include the psychological changes associated with puberty and, to a lesser extent, with menopause and aging.

Such a concept of development is, therefore, often very useful for understanding human growth and functioning. However, the concept becomes too constrictive, and at times truly inapplicable, when we attempt to apply it to all aspects of continuing growth and development in adults. Here it seems less reasonable to attribute development in every case to an underlying biological thrust.

In comparison, the following definition of development is more applicable to many experiences of adult life, including that of being seriously ill:

> A crisis of development occurs when an individual experiences significant internal change, external change, or both. The result is an initial phase of awareness, during which the individual struggles with the wish to know that he has changed versus the wish not to know. This is followed by a phase of disorganization, as the individual experiences a breakdown in his previously established homeostasis. There is then a phase of resolution as the individual begins to establish a new internal organization, a new relationship to external reality, or both. The changes that a given individual effects are always motivated by a basic need to restore homeostasis. When the changes result in regression, constriction of human potential, and withdrawal of interest in the future, we can speak of a *failure of mastery*. When, on the other hand, the changes lead to progress, expansion of human potential, and renewed investment in the future, we can speak of *mastery* or *development*. (DER)

One can think of many stunning instances in which people have mastered their illness and continued to grow considerably. Examples range from Franklin D. Roosevelt to Abraham Lincoln (who probably had Marfan's syndrome) to Helen Keller.

Obviously, the vast majority of our patients respond to illness in ways that are less dramatic but no less real. The dignity and grace that Mrs. Clark displays in Chapter 1 are not spectacular, yet they epitomize the capacity that many patients have to martial qualities of wisdom and bravery in the face of severe illness. Conversely, the businessman who, after a heart attack, quietly, gradually, gives up his interest in sex, then in his business, and finally in life may well go unnoticed. We may notice only that his EKG has improved and his enzymes returned to normal. His vital signs are improved, but his vitality is dead. Too often we heal the organ, but not the spirit.

THE THREE STAGES OF ILLNESS

Looked at from a developmental perspective, significant illness can be conceptualized as having three stages:
1. Awareness
2. Disorganization
3. Reorganization

Individuals may or may not progress through all three stages. That will depend primarily on the severity and chronicity of the illness. Stage one, awareness, is characterized by *ambivalence about knowing*. During this phase, an individual begins to realize that something is wrong. In some way his body or his mind is not working the way it should. It is a phase of increasing anxiety and bewilderment, as the patient struggles to deny and minimize his symptoms on the one hand and seeks to gain an understanding and explanation for them on the other. Many illnesses never progress beyond stage one. From time to time we all develop a fever, a lump, or a bump. The thought may cross our minds, "Is this cancer? Am I dying?" "No," we will respond. "It's just a bump. It's just a bruise." Usually this turns out to be true, the symptoms abate, and the whole episode, including the brief glimpse of mortality that it imposes, is entirely forgotten.

If the illness does not go away, the patient will progress to stage two. During this stage, many profound changes occur, but above all there is a *shattering of omnipotence*. The patient can no longer deny that something is wrong. This disrupts a universal defense—the magical belief that somehow we are immune from disease, injury, and death. Cancer always happens to someone else. It's always just a name in a newspaper when someone gets hit and killed by a bus. With the shattering of omnipotence, other major alterations occur in the way that the individual perceives his relationship to himself, to other people, and to reality itself.

If the illness does not resolve spontaneously or lead to rapid death, the patient will enter stage three, reorganization. During this stage, the patient responds to the changes that have been forced upon him. He alters his view of himself, of others, and of reality. In short, he changes. The goal of all change during this period is homeostasis, the re-establishing of equilibrium. The re-establishing of homeostasis may be regressive or progressive, growth constricting or growth promoting. The outcome of stage three will typically depend on the resources available to the patient—the resources within himself that he brings to the experience and the resources around him, including family, lovers, and friends—and, last but not least, the nature of his relationship to his doctor.

Awareness

Ambivalence About Knowing

As Cassell has pointed out, a person can have a disease without being ill. In order to be ill, a person must know he is sick. Thus, someone suffering from silent hypertension has a disease; but, if he is without symptoms and is not aware of his hypertension, he is not ill. Illness, then, is more than pathophysiology and diseased tissue. Rather, it is a drastic alteration, brought on by sickness, in an individual's relationship to reality and to his sense of identity.

Nor does the severity of illness always correlate with the degree of disease pathology alone. Just as the silent hypertensive may not be ill at all, the cardiac cripple whose heart functioning is excellent but whose relationship to life has become drastically constricted is very ill. Certain kinds of disease, by their symbolism alone, create symptoms of severe illness. In our culture, with its dread of cancer, a person is apt to feel, at some level, that he is literally being eaten alive, even if the cancer has a good prognosis.

The first stage of illness begins, then, when a person becomes aware that something in his health seems to be going wrong. The threshold of this awareness varies and depends on many factors, including the nature of the symptoms. A person is far more likely to ignore a painless swelling than the sudden onset of rectal bleeding.

Initially, there may be only puzzlement. There comes a point, however, where the symptoms can no longer be dismissed. At this point, the individual experiences an intense conflict between his wish to know what is wrong and his dread of knowing what is wrong—*ambivalence about knowing*.

Why not use the more common expression, *denial?* The answer is that the latter term fails to capture the conflicted nature of the experience. Denial is only half the conflict. Most of us *want* to know as badly as we want not to know. Early in an illness, especially, patients invariably feel two strongly opposing pulls about how much they really want to find out.

Some patients claim they want everything disclosed—"Tell it like it is." Others seem to beseech, in countless ways, against being told anything—"It's in your hands, doctor, I'm sure you'll do what's best." It is a mistake, however, to overlook the unexpressed half of any patient's ambivalence. Thus, the person who bravely wants you to "tell all" may secretly dread hearing the truth. To state the realities to him too baldly, too soon, may cause depression, despair, and giving up. Conversely, the patient who says, "It's up to you, doc," still may need some explanation of what's going on.

This vacillation can often lead to some very odd bargains that patients strike with reality. Sometimes these can go on for a surprisingly long time.

Mr. Bedford was a 55-year-old business executive with early alcoholic cirrhosis. The first symptoms were mild enlargement of his breast tissue, some very annoying and intractible hemorrhoids, and an occasional tendency for his eyes to turn a bit yellow. At one level, Mr. Bedford knew what was going on. He was educated enough to know especially that jaundice was associated with liver disease. He also knew, at least every morning when he woke up with a hangover, that he drank too much. On more than one occasion, he had resolved to see a doctor. Yet, for a number of months, he found ways to dismiss the symptoms. He began to work out in a gym because "my chest is getting flabby." He tried a variety of remedies for his hemorrhoids, which he attributed to constipation. At one point, he resorted to taking sunlamp treatments in an attempt to mask his jaundice from himself. He finally sought medical attention many months later when his abdomen began to swell from ascites and he could no longer rationalize this as "just putting on a little weight."

One can see here how overly simplistic it would be to reduce everything that Mr. Bedford did to denial. Certainly he was denying. Yet, his actions also reflect the other side of his ambivalence. On occasion he thought of going to a doctor. There were several periods where he "cut back" because

"I know the booze is bad for me." In addition he implemented a number of quasi-medical self-treatments. While these were designed to cover up his illness, they were also reflections of his knowledge that he was getting sick.

Ambivalence about knowing is not diminished by a person's level of education. In fact, doctors and medical students are often the most flagrant examples of this ambivalence. Everyone knows the story of at least one physician who denied obvious warning signals of disease, using his medical knowledge to rationalize and avoid the truth. I displayed this in my own illness.

Another example of this ambivalence within our profession is the medical student's so-called "hypochondriasis." The term is actually misleading. True hypochondriacs tend to relish their symptoms and need them in order to feel secure, no matter how much they complain. What medical students experience is not hypochondriasis but a terrifying anxiety about their own vulnerability, brought on by constant exposure to illness and death. During episodes of intense anxiety about disease, these students will often seem to be displaying an unambivalent wish to know, yet their dread of knowing is usually just below the surface.

> Janet, a junior medical student on orthopaedics, had some pain in her right knee. Convinced that she had developed an osteosarcoma, she spent several days feeling thoroughly certain that she was soon to die from a painful, disfiguring disease. After three days of this anguish, she went to an orthopaedist.
>
> The orthopaedist had his nurse take some x-rays of the affected area before he began his examination. Ten or 20 minutes later when he entered the examining room, he greeted Janet with a cheery "Hi!"
>
> Janet, upon hearing this word, immediately gasped, burst into tears and exclaimed, "You mean it's already gone into my thigh?!"

Turning Inward

Early in the course of an illness, an individual finds himself turning inward and becoming increasingly self-absorbed. Early in my own illness, there were many occasions when I would attempt to concentrate on matters outside myself, trying to pay attention to teaching rounds at the hospital, trying to watch TV without drifting off, or trying to read a book. But always my thoughts would slowly drift back toward my symptoms, toward myself. One experiences a sense of preoccupation and irritability, a self-centeredness that is monotonous and frightening, yet somehow inescapable. It feels, in a way, as if life has become a TV set, stuck on one channel, tuned to a program that is abhorred yet that cannot be turned off.

A subtle sense of disconnectedness from others begins to set in. Contradictory feelings about closeness appear, often with startling intensity. Two conflicts are especially common: the conflict between dependence and independence and the conflict between dread of separation and the longing for withdrawal.

Dependence Versus Independence. It is common to say of patients that they fight becoming dependent. This is certainly true—part of the time.

It is equally common to hear how illness causes a person to become dependent, demanding, clinging, and regressed. This is also true—part of the time. Often, we hear these reactions being attributed to different "personality types."

Doubtless, such people exist, and the notion of personality types is useful. However, for most of us, it is more accurate to say that we usually feel two ways about dependence at once: the typical patient vacillates between a wish to remain independent and a longing to be taken care of. I displayed this conflict during my own illness. On the one hand, I would go to great lengths to assert my independence. I refused for quite a while to allow anyone to treat me as sick. I prided myself on my ability to continue my duties as a medical student and, especially, my ability to hide my suffering from others. I saw any sign of "weakness" in myself as a kind of disgrace. Such an attitude defied reason, of course, but it is extremely common, especially among men.

Simultaneously, my behavior would be completely the opposite. This, incidentally, is another characteristic of altered thinking in illness: paradoxes and contradictions that would ordinarily feel entirely illogical come to be accepted as comn onplace. Thus, even as I struggled to maintain a stance of "bravery" and independence, I clearly was regressed, dependent, and at times fanatically insistent about my right to certain indulgences. In many subtle and not so subtle ways, I expected my wife to wait on me hand and foot. Moreover, at entirely unpredictable moments I would expect her to display great sympathy and understanding, even though a few hours previously I had barked at her for doing just that.

How can such contradictory emotions and behavior exist in the same person? It seems true beyond argument that under extreme stress—and illness is such a stress—all of us have a tendency to revert to earlier, more child-like ways of thinking about ourselves and perceiving the world. This is precisely what happens in the case of the sick person. As children, most of us were once highly dependent on our parents. And as the stress of illness begins to encroach on us, we re-experience with heightened vividness struggles and longings that originated in our childhood. On the one hand, we are scared. We feel helpless, uncertain, and small; we long for safety and reassurance. It is not so much the dependency itself that we yearn for as it is the sense of security that goes with it. Yet, as these longings emerge, and we feel ourselves slipping back, we discover that we have purchased one kind of security at the cost of another. To feel dependent and little again threatens our sense of competence, self-sufficiency, and control. If we allow ourselves to feel dependent, we fear that we will have to relinquish our grasp on all the security that comes from being an adult, the security that we have in our strength, autonomy, and self-sufficiency.

Thus, the person who is becoming ill finds himself oscillating between two equally untenable solutions. If he remains a self-sufficient adult, he feels deeply frightened and alone. If he gives in to dependent longings in an attempt to capture the security that comes from being taken care of, he relinquishes his sense of autonomy, self-sufficiency, and independence. As a result, the typical patient shows every sign of constantly being at war between these two solutions.

Dread of Separation Versus Longing for Withdrawal. In a similar way, a person who is becoming ill often experiences great conflicts over being alone. On the one hand, an acutely ill person longs for a lack of stimulation. One discerns a distinct wish to be left alone, as though to withdraw inward, conserving strength and husbanding energy.

Yet, one also sees the opposite, a fear of being alone, sometimes bordering on panic, for aloneness also symbolizes separation, vulnerability, and even the threat of death. To appreciate how universal and deep-seated is the connection between aloneness and the fear of death, one need only think of the many contemporary suspense films based on this theme, e.g., *Psycho* (directed by Hitchcock), *Wait Until Dark* (Young), and *Klute* (Pakula).

In my view, the longing for aloneness that occurs early in illness is not readily explained. It is possible, of course, to attribute a symbolic significance to it; but early in the course of illness, there seems to be an almost physical aversion to excessive stimulation, whether it be sensory (bright lights, loud noises, strong smells) or emotional (intense feelings). Perhaps the brain's response to incoming stimuli is altered; with a massive influx of somatic stimuli signaling physical distress, it seems plausible that the brain responds by selectively filtering out and reducing other kinds of stimuli as a mode of self-protection.

Dread of separation, on the other hand, is highly symbolic and readily understood as a powerful threat of aloneness, helplessness, and death. It may conceivably have its deepest origins in the experience of helplessness and dependence that we all felt as infants. Whatever the ultimate psychological and physiological antecedents may be, the ill person usually finds himself torn between his longing for closeness and his need to withdraw.

Fighting Change

When an individual becomes seriously ill, he experiences a major disruption in everything that moors him to life. Ties to reality, to other people, and ultimately to his sense of self are all severely strained. The rupturing of these ties and the individual's attempts to re-establish them comprise the major developmental task of being ill. Early on, however, a patient will typically react to such disruption by trying to retain an older, outmoded sense of himself; he will try, sometimes desperately, to hang onto the fantasy that he has not changed.

THE FRACTURING OF TIME

The moving finger writes; and, having writ,
Moves on; not all your piety nor wit
Shall lure it back to cancel half a line
Nor all your tears wash out a word of it.
                    The Rubáiyát of Omar Kháyyám

Not long ago, I was awakened in my home around 1:00 a.m. by loud knocking at the front door. When I answered it, I found one of my neighbors, still dressed in evening clothes, visibly frightened and holding back tears. She told me that she was worried about her husband, whom she feared had had a heart attack. They had been out at the theater. After the show, during a late supper, her husband had begun to complain first of indigestion and then chest pain. Could I take a look?

One look at Mr. Pennington, and I suspected that his wife's worst fears were real. He was lying on the sofa, his shirt collar unbuttoned and his tie pulled askew. His complexion was pale and I could see that he was perspiring profusely. His pulse was 120. I began to make arrangements to call an ambulance immediately.

At this point, however, Mr. Pennington began to protest. Couldn't we put it off? The pain seemed to be subsiding. He *couldn't* go to the hospital tonight. Mr. Pennington was a CPA. Tomorrow morning at 8:00 sharp he had to be present at an audit of an important client. Furthermore, that afternoon, he had another important meeting that couldn't possibly be cancelled. "Couldn't we delay this whole thing for 24 hours, doc?"

Mr. Pennington was displaying one of the most common early reactions to illness, the struggle to hang on to a pre-illness sense of time. Physicians repeatedly run into this—patients in the emergency room who "just have to go home" to attend to a few overlooked chores or patients with important plans for the following day that can't possibly be cancelled. These patients are fighting to hang on to the most important connections that moor them to their sense of identity: their past, their present, and above all, their future. Later in the course of illness, patients experience a profound disruption of their moorings in time. They experience themselves as irrevocably, undeniably changed; they can no longer reconcile an outmoded image of themselves, with all its memories and plans, with their greatly altered present reality. Early in the course of illness, however, the disruption will be seen most conspicuously, and often very poignantly, in a wish to hang on to the future. It is as though these patients find it inconceivable that tomorrow will dawn any differently from the way they had planned.

When a patient wants to leave the emergency room abruptly or sign out of the hospital AMA (against medical advice), his behavior seems so destructive and irrational to most physicians that the patient usually comes in for his share of anger. Yet, often such patients are struggling to hang onto their future—and their sense of who they are—which they feel being wrenched away from them by their illness.

Threat to the Physical Self. Most of us take our bodies for granted. When we want to go, we go. If we need to run to catch a bus, we can. For most of us, the body is a remarkable, highly forgiving machine that responds to one's wishes and tolerates occasional abuses and excesses. Obviously, in any significant illness, our sense of physical integrity is disrupted. Even a minor cold can make one feel out of touch, and anything more serious tends to wreak havoc.

Our earliest identity is a body identity. We are introduced to the world through the sensations in our mouths and bellies as infants. We know hunger, sucking, and relief from hunger. We learn warmth and cold, wet and dry. As we grow, locomotion becomes the all important medium of self-awareness—reaching for an object, rolling over, sitting up, and finally walking. Thus, our earliest experiences in development create a self-definition that is fundamentally physical. The bodily origins of our sense of self show up in many aspects of our thinking, including our language. We say, "I just won't *stand* for that." "How are you going to *handle* that situation?" In thinking, we *reach* a conclusion. When we have trouble, we *run up against* a problem. When we figure something out, we *grasp* it. In other words, even our later mental representations of thinking and abstraction are often rooted in our bodily sense of ourselves.

The reaction of a person to the threatened loss of physical integrity can be powerful and irrational. I recall driving once on a mountain road behind two young men on a motorcycle. Going around a curve, they hit a patch of gravel and dropped the bike. They slid for literally hundreds of feet, pinned under the bike. Finally, the bike came to a stop and I pulled up behind them. Before I had a chance to prevent it, one of them hopped to his feet, covered with gravel and blood, and began walking in circles saying "I'm alive, I'm alive, I'm alive." From an orthopaedic standpoint, getting up after a possible spinal injury was tantamount to suicide. From a psychological standpoint, it made perfect sense. This young man, frightened and hurt but still conscious, wanted to reassure himself that he was still literally in one piece. He did this by proving to himself that his body was still all there and could still follow commands. He could get up, walk, and move his arms and legs. This was reassurance that he still existed.

Recall the two dreams I described during my own illness; a similar phenomenon will be discerned. In both dreams a specific wish is fulfilled—my bodily integrity is intact again. In the first dream, I am walking. In the second dream, I am swimming. The fact that each dream turns into a nightmare says something about the strong unconscious relationship between illness and a threat to bodily integrity. This is especially clear in the second dream, in which I am pursued by a shark.

Irrational, idiosyncratic behavior connected with the body is one of the most common, early symptoms of a person's struggle with physical illness. Almost everyone has a favorite ritual—vitamin C, cold showers, hot showers, or exercise. It is distressingly common to see coronary victims attempt to cope with the onset of chest pain by resorting to vigorous activity and exercise. Many of us engage in at least some degree of magical thinking. "If I do A, then I can undo B." For some, the magical equation is exercise and body-building. For others, it can be health food, fad diets, or vitamins. The affinity that many otherwise rational people have for faith healers, charletons, and quacks may come from the fact that many of these quacks have more insight than physicians often have into the underlying anxiety of patients about loss of physical integrity.

Disorganization

The Shattering of Omnipotence

Once upon a time, a poor man and his wife had 12 children. When the 13th, a son, was born, the mother and father refused to bless him. The bitter father refused to allow God to be the Godfather. The Devil also offered to be his Godfather and was refused.

Finally, only Death came to the christening, and he alone agreed to bless this 13th child, and to be his Godfather.

"When you grow up," Death said, "You shall be a physician. I will give you the power to know who shall live and who shall die. When you are called to a patient's bedside, I shall stand at the head of the bed or the foot of the bed. If I stand at the head of the bed, the patient will die. If I stand at its foot, you can rest assured, the patient will live."

And thus the prophesy came to pass. The boy grew up to be a physician and the word of his skills spread far and wide. He was the most powerful, wealthy, sought after physician in the land.

One day, he was summoned to the bedside of the ailing king. To the physician's horror, Death came and stood at the head. In a quandary, the physician hesitated for a moment and then spun the bed around so that Death now stood at the foot. The king went on to recover.

"I shall forgive you this one time," Death told the physician. "But if you ever do it again, I shall strip you of your powers and your life."

The grateful physician agreed never to repeat his transgression.

Many years later the physician was again summoned to the king's castle. This time the king's only daughter, a fair beautiful princess, lay ill. One look and the physician fell in love. Death came, however, and once again stood at the head of the bed.

And once again, in spite of himself, the physician spun the bed around so that Death stood at its foot.

This time, Death did not forgive the physician. Despite his pleading, Death angrily spirited him away to a cave. There the physician beheld thousands of candles of different lengths, each burning slowly down in the darkness.

"Each of these candles represents a life," Death said. "When they burn down, a person's life is ended."

Death showed the physician his own candle. It had burned down to the very base, and was now little more than a tiny flicker.

"Please give me just one more chance!" implored the physician.

"It cannot be done," said Death, with a steely voice.

Slowly, Death reached out his finger and snuffed the physician's candle, once so bright.

My version of "Godfather Death," A Grimms' Fairy Tale (DER)

This fairytale makes many interesting points, not the least of which is the connection between a wish for control over death and the choice of physicianhood as a career. It is included here to illustrate a universal and ancient longing in all of us, the wish for omnipotence and for the most cherished aspect of omnipotence, immortality.

Not only do we wish for omnipotence, we spend a great deal of our normal waking lives functioning as though we actually possessed it. Philosophers and artists as diverse as Ernest Becker and Woody Allen have made the point repeatedly: denial of death seems to be one of the central features of our civilization, indeed of our very humanness.

There can be no doubt that, in normal functioning, we behave as though we are invulnerable. If we did not believe we were omnipotent, we probably would not get behind the wheel of a car, much less get on a freeway, much less drive a motorcycle or hangglide. We certainly wouldn't smoke cigarettes.

The sense of omnipotence with which we conduct our lives seems essential. It appears to function as a kind of psychological ectoplasm that gives us security and a sense of cohesiveness. It is almost as though we fear that the unruly cytoplasm of our deepest anxieties would spill out in a thousand directions if such a magical membrane did not exist. Some of us feel more secure in this omnipotence than others, but even the most conservative and timid among us possesses this fantasy most of the time.

The origins of our belief in our own omnipotence may reside in childhood. During a certain phase of their development, children idealize their parents, attributing to them godlike capacities and the absolute ability to protect them from all harm. Few children have not had the experience of being afraid of going to sleep at night, especially in a dark room. Fears of monsters, bogeymen, and kidnappers at the window are universal. Clearly, children at times perceive the world as a dangerous, inhospitable place. Typically, they derive security from the thought that mommy and daddy are in the next room and therefore can protect them from harm. At a later stage of development this fantasy of benevolent protection and omnipotence, originally externalized and attributed to the parents, becomes internalized. Thus, each of us as adults has a belief that some guiding force will keep us from harm. We all secretly harbor the fantasy that "it can't happen to me," that we lead a charmed life.

As Cassell has observed, the shattering of omnipotence is a major response to becoming seriously ill. I regard it as the central indicator that a patient has moved from stage one of illness into stage two, Disorganization.

The patient who has struggled to forestall his awareness of serious illness and then has finally recognized the truth is one of the most fragile, defenseless, and exquisitely vulnerable people one can ever find. This is a time of terror and depression.

Depending on the personality of the individual whose sense of omnipotence has been shattered, feelings of shame, lowered self-esteem, and guilt can also be present. In different patients, the central symbolism varies. For some individuals, serious illness may be proof that, in some mysterious way, they have sinned. For certain, especially self-sufficient people, the dependency of illness may be deeply humiliating and shattering. Whatever the particular symbolism, however, there is a clear commonality: significant illness disrupts a person's sense of invulnerability and omnipotence and shatters his sense of intactness. This will invariably result in turmoil, anxiety, and psychological disruption—a stage of disorganization.

Loss of Connection

No man is an island

John Donne

One of the features of our medical system that often leads to a misunderstanding of our patients is the practice of attending to patients only in offices, clinics, or hospitals. From this limited perspective, we may easily fail to appreciate the rich matrix of relationships, activities, beliefs, and interests that define people and give meaning to their lives. Too often we see only supine figures, stripped of their clothing, stripped of their world, looking up at us from a hospital bed.

Hospitals, offices, waiting rooms, receptionists, partitions, and double doorways with no admittance signs—all of these serve a real purpose. They make our work as doctors more comfortable psychologically, and they give us quick access to the tools of diagnosis and treatment that we need. They also cut our patients off from the world they live in and make it easy for us to neglect the humanness of the people we treat.

Early in the course of an illness, a patient finds his thoughts and preoccupations turning inward, away from people, often very much in spite of himself. As the illness progresses, this sense of disconnectedness from people becomes ever more pronounced. In hospitalized patients, the separation, in fact, is virtually absolute. People are wrenched from their jobs, from their bedrooms, from their favorite robes and slippers and from their families, coffee cups, books, pipes, and favorite pictures on the wall. They are thrust into an alien world of bright lights, beeping electric monitors, tubes, tangles of wires, and strangers. The effect can be shattering. More than one patient has signed out of the hospital against medical advice because the separation seemed unbearable. The austerity and alienation of modern hospitals does raise the question, is all of this impersonality really necessary for the sake of efficiency, or are we needlessly isolating patients from what is loved and familiar, what connects them to life itself?

For most patients, however, psychological separation is far more traumatic than physical separation. Even without a hospital, illness produces awesome separation. Consider the view our culture traditionally holds toward persons with tuberculosis and leprosy. Despite the fact that both are treatable and no longer highly contagious diseases, they continue to elicit a certain irrational dread, and we regard people suffering from them as outcasts. Indeed, the word "leper" has come to mean outcast in our vocabulary. Occasionally this isolation has been romanticized, as in Thomas Mann's *The Magic Mountain*, or used as a political allegory, as in Solzhenitsyn's *The Cancer Ward.* The cruel fact is, such isolation is seldom romantic for the patient. It is grim and depressing. Until very recently, the mentally ill were housed in asylums far from population centers. Now they are back in our communities. But are they outcasts any the less?

Patients often impose isolation upon themselves—an isolation far more fearsome than physical separation alone would be. This occurred in my own illness. In the first of my two dreams, for example, my isolation from people is clearly symbolized. I am at the bottom of a deep well, perhaps a symbol for a grave, looking up at the sky—at life—calling to people I love. Yet when one of them tries to reach me, I experience dread. If she joins me, she too may be afflicted with my curse.

The notion of "catching," in fact, is surprisingly widespread. I once worked with a middle-aged couple; the wife had cancer. Although neither of them would initially say so, both finally admitted to an embarrassing fantasy: the husband was afraid he would catch his wife's cancer, and the wife was afraid that she might pass this curse to her husband, especially if they had physical contact. As a result, they had ceased completely to have sexual relations. In fact, her cancer was in good remission and her prognosis was excellent, but reality does not automatically rid people of their deepest fears.

Many times, such patients turn to the physician, who may represent the only person who can commute freely back and forth across the ever widening breach that separates the sick from the well, a separation that exists mostly in the mind, but one far more deadly than any that a mere physical barrier could impose.

Shattering of Identity

When the Body Fails. In health, we take our bodies for granted. In disease, the body becomes a prison. Normally, we aren't aware of our constant breathing. For the person with emphysema, each gasp becomes a battle between the relentless hunger for air and the unceasing pain of failing lungs. In health, we do not notice our hearts. For the postcoronary patient, each beat is a reaffirmation of life and every change a potential death knell.

In a sense, the patient becomes his body. The horizons of his life shrink until all that remain are aches, pains, and symptoms. He *is* a diseased heart. He has *become* emphysema. The ill person does not welcome this narrowness; but he simply cannot help it.

Listen to the talk of an old person whose health has begun to fail. It is filled with references to bowel function, diet, joint pain, and medication. Such preoccupations can seem boring, signs of a doddering senility. In fact, they are evidence of a vigil. The ill person is watching himself ever more closely, attending more and more to each little change in his body. Consciousness can, and sometimes does, narrow to a tremor, to a twinge of pain, to the beat of a heart.

This narrowness of vision is not exclusive to hospitalized patients. For the individual who has left the hospital, life may still become a maze of inconveniences, hazards, and restrictions centered around his illness. Will he have to climb steps? Will there be a place to rest? What happens if he runs out of nitroglycerin? Will he be near a bathroom? Will he soil?

It is hard to overestimate the impact that this distortion of a person's daily reality begins to have. A previously healthy person finds himself changed from someone with a wide variety of interests and involvements into a prisoner, a captive to his own physiology, constantly vigilant to every real or imagined change in body function. Reality has shrunk to a matter of pulse rate and breath.

Discontinuity of the Self. We are not just bodies, however, and the ill person feels himself losing something even more cherished than his sense of physical wholeness. With illness comes a devastating loss of the sense of self.

We maintain our sense of integration as individuals through a variety of channels. These include our beliefs, accomplishments, and ideals; our surroundings, tastes, and the food we eat; the work we do, the friends we have;

our memories and our plans. Among these and others that help to comprise our sense of self, an absolutely critical landmark is our sense of continuity in time. The origins of discontinuity in time can be seen early in illness, especially in the tendency people have to cling to the future. As illness advances, a profound rupturing of continuity occurs. Patients feel they have lost something in their bodies to be sure; but, beyond this, they have also lost important symbols of continuity in time. The awareness dawns that they are no longer who they used to be. The past is gone. The future is uncertain. Plans must be modified or even abandoned.

The struggles that patients undergo around this loss can be quite intense. Recall Mrs. Clark in Chapter 1. When Paul walks in to her hospital room, he finds her bald, yet holding a mirror and a brush. After some initial embarrassment, she finally says, "You caught me with the brush this morning. It's just that when I first wake up each morning, sometimes I forget—well, no . . . that's not true. The truth is that sometimes I *pretend*. I say to myself, 'Today I'll look in the mirror and I'll be a beautiful young woman again . . . '"

In a sense, illness shatters memory. Suddenly, we are no longer what we were. For many patients, this can feel almost as though life were a cherished scrap book filled with old clippings and photographs, but on every page Illness, the censor, has left his imprint in huge red letters—VOID.

Pause for a moment and think about your own sense of memory. Think back to an early memory, one from childhood, perhaps ages 5 to 10. As you do so, you'll find that you can feel what it was like then. In fact, you feel like the same person you are today. It was you then, just as it is you now. At a gut level there is the sensation of sameness and continuity. If you think about this for a moment, it is really quite remarkable. Consider how much you have actually changed—physically, psychologically, in all respects of your life—since then. Yet, you feel like the same person. This is because, in some very complicated way, we normally develop a coherent sense of self; and a great deal of this sense of continuity rests on our feeling of sameness over time. We think of ourselves as evolving, yet having a core that is stable and enduring which does not change over time. Illness invariably threatens to disrupt this sense, and people react with great anxiety.

A moving portrayal of the struggle around loss of self is contained in the film, *Brian's Song*, the true story of a young football player named Brian Piccolo who was stricken in his 20s with lung cancer. In the drama, Brian goes through an initial stage of awareness, during which he struggles to accept the truth, followed by a stage of disorganization. He begins to realize that he may never play football again. He is frail where he once was strong. He is losing weight. Yet, he still struggles to retain his sense of identity as an athlete. At one point, he plaintively says, "Maybe I can still be a kicker. You don't need much wind for that." Clearly, what he has lost goes beyond bodily health. He has lost the sense of who he is. And he must now begin the struggle of redefining who he will be.

Ultimately, a patient's task will be to integrate new realities into a suddenly outmoded self-perception, to establish once again a sense of connectedness to the future. Initially, most patients understandably feel devastated and bitter. Memories are cruel, tantalizing the patient, filling him with yearning for an irretrievable past. The future seems nonexistent. During this stage, significant depression is common.

The loss of a continuous sense of self is always shattering. It can be especially shattering, however, when the illness encroaches on the parts of our self that we prize most. It is understandable that loss of lung capacity would feel especially cruel to Brian Piccolo. It seems diabolical that Beethoven went deaf. Symptoms of central nervous dysfunction—loss of memory, disorientation, hallucinations—are, as Cassell has observed, especially devastating. He points out that these are person-symptoms, whereas many illnesses cause body-symptoms. This is what devastated young Arrowsmith in the Sinclair Lewis novel by that name: that his beloved teacher, Professor Gottlieb, could become ill might be acceptable, but that this brilliant man would lose his mind to senility tore Arrowsmith apart. For many of us, being unable to think is the most fearsome loss of all.

Distortions in Thinking

During illness, a patient's mode of thinking about reality will often undergo mysterious, frightening changes and distortions. Thinking becomes increasingly idiosyncratic, self-centered, and at times even reveals some belief in magic.

Superstition. People normally accustomed to conducting their lives with balance and rationality may frequently find themselves becoming mildly superstitious.

"I took those aspirin an hour ago and now the tremor in my left hand seems less."

"My stomach feels better than it ever has since I ate that oatmeal."

People find themselves grasping at any small straw, any causal connection between a slight improvement in symptoms and some act of omission or commission that they can control.

Some people, who otherwise function at an entirely rational level, become overtly superstitious. One patient felt compelled to tap five different locations in his bathroom three times each morning. He knew that this procedure would not really help his arthritis, but he felt compelled to perform it nonetheless.

One woman, a 45-year-old telephone operator dying of cancer, clung to a worn paperback entitled *The Grape Cure* until the very end. This book offered her a magical solution to a seemingly insoluble problem. Ordinarily, she would not have been susceptible to the distortions of reality that accepting the book's premise required. In the height of her illness, she found herself drawn to these distortions.

The vulnerability of ill people to belief in magic is, at one level, quite understandable. Just as primitive cultures often invoke mystical explanations for natural phenomena that seem incomprehensible and frightening, magical thinking offers some promise of coherence and order in the face of chaos. The wish for this cuts very deep. Many physicians no doubt contribute unwittingly to some of their patients' decisions to turn to quackery. The physician who cannot empathize with his patients, who speaks cryptically or tersely and does not provide adequate explanations, may be inviting them to seek coherence and reassurance elsewhere.

Egocentrism. Beyond superstition, another common change in the ill person's mode of thinking is egocentrism. There is a great tendency among people who suffer from illness to begin to see themselves as far more central to the world than is justified or than they would ordinarily view themselves. Many ill people become hypersensitive to the behavior of those around them. If a nurse is 10 minutes late with a sleeping pill, such patients will be convinced that she does not like them or is angry at them for some imagined, earlier transgression. The families of such people also come in for considerable flack. A wife who is late for a visit or is moody or preoccupied will be accused of "being angry at me"—"What did I do?!" The sick person is often drawn to a position from which he looks out and sees himself as responsible for everything around him.

This phenomenon is less mysterious if we realize that, like many other seemingly puzzling behaviors, it has its origins in thinking and reasoning that were normal during childhood. In many ways, in spite of his efforts, the ill person will feel himself to be a child. He will often react to people who take care of him and love him more as parents than as equals. The result is a tendency toward self-centeredness and demandingness that the patient often finds embarrassing, yet cannot resist. This is what I was displaying in my own illness when I ranted and raved at my wife for kicking over the typewriter. I had regressed to a position in which she was my mother, and the world centered around me, my needs, and my wishes. When these were thwarted, I felt frustrated, furious, and afraid.

Guilt. Another manifestation of egocentrism can be guilt. It is surprisingly common for patients to believe, at some level, that their illness is a punishment for some transgression. This idea is as deeply entrenched for many people as it is embarrassing and unexpressible. Many religious systems do, in fact, equate illness with punishment for sin. A modern day derivative is the tendency of many sophisticated patients to accuse themselves of being "psychosomatic." This is what I did in my illness; it is very common among doctors in general. Such patients often have a difficult time quite believing that they are sick at all and will constantly ruminate—"Did I bring this on myself? Am I exaggerating? Is it emotional?" The questions do not emanate from a real desire to understand the connections between disease and psychological distress. Rather, they are subtle expressions of guilt, of the unconscious notion that the patient is somehow responsible for bringing on his own downfall. It may be that some of us find this notion, as painful as it is, less traumatic than the idea that our illness could be due to chance, entirely random, and therefore totally beyond our control.

Shame. Some patients may also show an unreasonable self-centeredness in the form of shame and embarrassment. The patient I mentioned above, who subscribed to the grape cure, was a very attractive woman who placed great emphasis on her physical appearance. She seemed especially preoccupied with the disfiguring effects of her cancer, even more than she was with her impending death. In fact, she did something that shocked me deeply when I first met her in an interviewing course as a freshman medical student. After giving me a few minutes of her history, she suddenly disrobed and exposed her cancerous breasts, inviting me to palpate them. At the time, I did not understood that her exhibitionism was the mirror opposite of her deep sense of shame. She was desperately seeking reassurance that her illness had not made her hideous.

Many men, especially, try to live up to a Gary Cooper stereotype, suffering silently and trying to hide their pain. Disclosure to them seems shameful. In my own illness, one of my strongest wishes was to make a good showing to the world, from the outset, when I tried to hide my cramping from my friends, to a later stage, when I took great pride in my ability to give a speech and to hide my physical distress. I had a deep need to show the world that I was tough and strong.

Despite differences in emphasis from person to person, the combination of withdrawal of interest in external reality, increasing preoccupation with internal bodily functions, and growing self-centeredness are almost universal. Furthermore, these changes are usually experienced as alarming symptoms in their own right. A patient will frequently express chagrin that he is "acting like a baby" or "can't seem to get it together." He senses his regression, yet is truly unable to fight it. Often, a patient will secretly believe that the changes in his thinking are sure evidence that he is going mad. Such anxiety, of course, compounds the apprehensions and sense of separation he already feels: not only is he different physically—on top of that he feels he is going crazy. The physician who makes a point of being alert to such concerns will find they are surprisingly common. A little bit of empathy and reassurance can go a long way toward relieving patients from this kind of suffering.

Loss of Autonomy

It's hard to forget Mr. Greenspoon. At 62, he is well known in local civic organizations and a key sponsor of the museum and opera company. A self-made man with a high school education, he parlayed a small hardware business into a vast fiscal conglomerate. He is a millionaire. He is also hypertensive, 50 pounds overweight, and excessively fond of cigars. He currently occupies a bed in the hospital to which he has made major donations. He is in for a gallbladder removal.

Initially, the nurses found him "cute," "a really funny guy." They found it amusing that first morning when he got caught smoking a huge cigar before breakfast. As the day wore on, however, his endless defiance of hospital routine quickly wore thin. At one point, they found him out at the nurses' desk, commandeering the phone lines. When asked to use his own bedside phone, he said he had to keep that free. He was waiting for an important call. He complained loudly about the food. He refused to have his i.v. inserted by the i.v. nurse and demanded that this simple procedure be performed by the head of surgery, whom, he hastened to add, "I know personally!"

By 5:00 that evening, the once "cute" Mr. Greenspoon has turned into an institutional sorespot—as the nursing staff put it bluntly and in unison, "a real pain!"

Mr. Greenspoon, like many patients, is finding the loss of autonomy that the sick role imposes unbearable. Because he is rich and a bit of a bully, the staff finds him more difficult to manage than the typical patient. But his behavior is in many ways quite typical.

It may be easier to understand our patient's dilemma if we compare it to the experience of medical school. Just as medical school seems to isolate the student, stripping him of his identity and sense of accomplishments, so does the enforced dependency and regimentation imposed by illness wreak similar havoc with the patient. If one can get past Mr. Greenspoon's obnoxiousness and empathize with him, it is clear that he has suffered severe losses simply by entering the hospital. He is, after all, "a self-made man," as he is fond of saying. Think about the implications of this phrase: he has done it all on his own. In fact, as his history comes out, one learns that his father died when Mr. Greenspoon was 12. He was the oldest son and quickly became the man of the house, caring for his mother, who was left penniless, and his two younger sisters.

The loss of autonomy he faces as a patient, therefore, is truly terrifying. It calls forth in him many dreaded memories. To lose autonomy, to become dependent, is tantamount in Mr. Greenspoon's mind with being 12 years old again, without a daddy, facing fearsome responsibilities alone.

Loss of autonomy is not restricted to hospitalization. During the course of his gallbladder surgery, Mr. Greenspoon will receive a hypertension workup. It will disclose essential hypertension and his internist will start him on a regimen of antihypertensive medications. In the ensuing months, Mr. Greenspoon will not take them. Despite his wife's perpetual nagging, he will skip doses. He will also continue to salt his food liberally, enjoy two martinis before dinner, and refuse to cut back on his cigars.

"Dammit!" he will bellow when confronted. "I do what I please! You can all go to the devil!"

Most patients will show their dismay less flamboyantly than does Mr. Greenspoon; yet, he is in many ways prototypical, and his reaction to loss of autonomy leads us directly to another reaction to illness—rebellion.

Rebellion

"Do not go gentle into that good night,
Old age should burn and rave at close of day;
Rage, rage against the dying of the light.

Dylan Thomas

Illness can evoke a sense of helpless rage. It feels terribly unfair. "Why me?" is a bitter question that many people ask. The worst part, for many, is the diabolic way this sense of unfairness is coupled with feelings of absolute impotence. Whom can one lash out against? Whom can one strike back at? Whom can one blame? This was, of course, the existential question that tormented Job. The fact that the unfairness is random, inexplicable, and due to fate may feel intolerable. For some people, frustration may lead to a period of rebellion.

This is beautifully dramatized in the film *Coming Home* (directed by Ashby). Early in the film, a young veteran named Luke is in a VA hospital, receiving acute care for paraplegia, the result of a war injury in Vietnam. He is a sullen, restive man, clearly depressed yet unapproachable. When nurses and other patients reach out to him, he pushes them away with sarcasm and scorn.

His anger erupts one morning when he is wheeling himself down the hall, prone on a gurney. The frustration and rage show on his face, yet he tries to remain contemptuous and controlled. A young woman, Sally Hyde, with whom he will later fall in love, is walking down the hall, about to apply for a volunteer job. She turns momentarily and bumps into his gurney. The impact shakes loose a catheter bag. It bursts open on the floor and both of them are spattered with his urine.

His rage, humiliation, and agony erupt. Careening wildly down the halls, he goes on a rampage smashing objects, smashing people, smashing anything he can. He is crazed, grief-stricken, savage, and pitiful. Eventually he has to be subdued, sedated, and restrained. Thus, ironically, his rebellion forces even greater helplessness upon him.

The following day, still tied to his bed in restraints, he has to be fed by a hospital aide. Quieter now, but still in a savage rage, he spits the food out and will not swallow.

For many, rebellion is not so extreme. It may be as subtle as a refusal to take one's pills as prescribed. It may be the timid, yet unmistakable stubof an elderly woman who refuses to cooperate actively in her physical rehabilitation. It may even be as quiet as a sigh, a sad impenetrable wall that some patients erect that says, "Try as you may, I won't let you in."

Physicians tend to be very intolerant of rebellion. It seems incomprehensible to many of us that a patient would refuse the pill or the exercise that would make him better. Often, our initial reaction is to try to reason the patient out of such foolishness. If the patient still refuses to cooperate, our reaction may then become one of derision and disgust. "Who cares—she doesn't even *want* to get better!"

If we can understand, however, that rebellion may be a patient's reaction to helplessness, our empathy may increase. Many patients, in a masked and sometimes self-destructive way, are fighting to gain some sense of coherence and control through their revolt, attempting to fight back and express their anger at what feels to them to be the terrible randomness of life.

Acceptance

The stage of disorganization typically comes to an end when the patient accepts the reality of his illness. A new self-image begins to emerge. This is often heralded by expressions such as "You can't go on pitying yourself forever" and "Sooner or later you have to accept it." Patients also begin to experience reconnectedness with time. They may begin to speak again of their past, grieving for what they used to be. They also reconnect with the future: they begin to anticipate the changes, adaptations, and adjustments that will be necessary. In a sense, they have taken their illness into themselves and said, "This is me." They no longer regard the illness as a foreign agent that has temporarily invaded them.

Whether the new equilibrium is growth promoting and progressive, or growth constricting and regressive, will depend on factors to be discussed below.

Reorganization

Mastery and Failure

This chapter began with a definition of development that included the possibility of success or failure. One must acknowledge that this is tricky ground. To imply that some people do better at handling their illnesses than others is to make a value judgment, no matter how carefully it is couched. There can be great hazard in this, especially for physicians. In my experience, doctors are especially prone to moralizing, typically when they are up against a problem that they can't control or understand. Too often, we judge our patients as a way of handling our own exasperation. Thus, people similar to us—intellectually or socioeconomically—are "good patients who "want" to get better. People who are very different from us or who have complex and intractable diseases, become "crocks," "turkeys," and "gomers." Students who have not yet heard these terms, will.

Given these hazards, it is still important to acknowledge that some people *do* cope better with their illnesses than others do, because a number of factors influence how well a patient will cope, including our effectiveness as physicians. It is always important to remember, however, that each patient is, in his way, doing the very best he can. Our task as physicians begins with our attempt to understand our patients, not judge them. If, from our empathy, a spirit of hope and collaboration can grow, all the better! If cure becomes possible, better still! But this does not always happen. We can always, however, strive to understand our patients, respect them, and appreciate the difficulties they face. The following examples—one of failure and one of success—are presented in this spirit.

Failure of Mastery. A vivid example of failure to master can be found in the Charles Dickens novel, *Great Expectations*. In the book, Pip encounters an elderly spinster, Miss Havisham. Miss Havisham suffers from psychosis. She lives in a world of delusions that protect her from an unbearable reality. In her dream world, time has stopped. Many years previously, when she was young, she was jilted on her wedding day, and the blow was intolerable. In one very poignant episode, she takes Pip into a large abandoned room. There, frozen in time, Pip beholds the decorations and accoutrements of a lavish wedding celebration. The table is set with the finest silver and china, though the linen table cloth is moth-eaten and riddled with holes. In the center, ensconced in a thick tangle of spider webs, is the rotted wedding cake, a collapsed pile of dust, long since forgotten by time, but remembered by Miss Havisham.

In her dream world, which has become her reality, she waits only for the appearance of her beloved groom. Clearly, Miss Havisham has constricted her human potential, withdrawn from life, and traded in reality for the solace that comes only from dreams.

Mastery. The triumph of mastery, and especially the importance of love in achieving that mastery, is movingly depicted in *Coming Home*. Luke, the tormented veteran described earlier, does not remain forever in his prison of frustration and rage. Gradually, he begins to fall in love with Sally, whom he at first so vigorously resisted. As his love for her grows, his sense of dignity and self-worth return. By the end of the film, he emerges with new strength and wisdom. In one scene, he chains himself to an armory gate to protest the war in which he was injured. In another, he speaks to a group of graduating high school students who are considering entering the military. Not only has he accepted his illness, he has transcended it. His paraplegia has become a powerful symbol for the expression of his principles and beliefs. While no one would have wished such a tragedy on him, it seems likely that he would not have achieved such stature and dignity in his life had he not become paralyzed. The bridge back for him lay, as it does for many people, in his capacity to re-establish deep loving ties with another human being.

Here, clearly, is a person who has changed in a way that led to progress, expansion of human potential, and renewed investment in the future. Such triumphs are not restricted to fiction.

Factors Affecting Mastery

Several factors will be critical in determining whether a patient regresses or grows during the stage of reorganization. These include: 1) the patient's capacity to react flexibly to change; 2) the severity and meaning of the illness; 3) the support system; and 4) the effectiveness of medical care.

The Patient's Capacity to React Flexibly to Change.

Mrs. Allport was 63 when she fell in the shower and broke her hip. A dependent woman, she had been taken care of by someone most of her life. As a child, she had been dependent on her mother, especially after her father died when she was 8. She did not date during high school until she met her husband at age 18, the first and only man she ever went out with. After the marriage, she transferred her dependency needs to him. Because she was afraid to drive, he took her everywhere. Because she was very sensitive to separation, he turned down several jobs that would have meant career advancement for him but which necessitated travel. She also lived within three blocks of her mother until her death.

Six months prior to her hip injury, Mrs. Allport's husband had died. She had not adjusted well, had become depressed, and had begun to drink, which was probably a factor in her fall.

The corrective surgery was effective and full restoration of function seemed likely. Full recovery did not occur, however. Despite major heroics on the part of her physical therapists, she continued to complain of pain and refused to give up her walker.

Eventually, she had to be placed in a nursing home where she continued to go downhill. Ten years later, Mrs. Allport remained unable to walk without the aid of her walker. In addition she had developed a scoliosis which, in turn, had begun to aggravate a previously mild emphysema. This in turn was causing recurring bouts of bacterial pneumonia.

Despite what had begun as an entirely curable illness, Mrs. Allport was dwindling away.

There was much in Mrs. Allport's earlier history to predict what happened. It is usually very helpful, when trying to understand patients, to consider their "track record." Illness, after all, is rarely the first major disruption in their lives. How patients have responded to the challenge of other developmental tasks will give clues to how they will respond now. How did they do in school? Have there been major losses in their lives? Financial reversals? Disappointments? The resilience and resourcefulness with which people have handled the past will usually say a great deal about how they are going to handle the future.

Also, if we are to be truly empathic, we must learn to accept and respect those patients who cannot grow and change. There will be many Mrs. Allports in our practices. It is important that we learn to understand the often momentous fears that hold some people back from change. These individuals, too, have their reasons for being as they are. We must not moralize about our patients. A patient whose life events have shaped him in a way that makes growth difficult is not a "bad" person. Those patients who can grow as people during illness bring us great joy in our work, but they are not more worthy as human beings.

Severity and Meaning of the Illness.

Even at age 76, Earl Gorham still cut a dashing figure. Six foot-two, lean and handsome, he had a devilish smile and a twinkle in his eye.

When Earl died, he was in the hospital for treatment of congestive heart disease. This had plagued him in recent years and required several admissions. He had always responded rapidly to treatment, however, and the prognosis for this hospitalization had been good.

Earl was a flamboyant man. During his lifetime he had been a successful jazz musician, artist, and entrepreneur. At one point he had been a national champion hydroplane racer. Despite many illnesses, he had remained a garrulous, outgoing man who loved people and loved life.

During this hospitalization, however, something new happened. Earl, who prided himself on his physical attractiveness and appeal to women, developed a bad case of herpes zoster, shingles. He was recovering uneventfully at the time from his congestive heart failure. The herpes infection distressed him greatly, however. Upon looking at his face in the mirror, seeing it covered with scales and eructations, he had shuddered and then became depressed.

"I can't stand to look at myself this way," he had said.

That night he died in his sleep.

Earl's shattering of omnipotence occurred around the loss of his physical attractiveness. A vigorous, bold man who had withstood many illnesses, he regarded his facial deformity as a sign of frailty, ugliness, and aging. He could not survive the blow.

Obviously, the severity and meaning of a patient's illness will be important in determining his capacity to adapt, as it was for Earl. Still, even in the most severe illness, one constantly encounters patients who discover resources they did not know they possessed. People can learn to live without limbs. Women can learn to accept mastectomies. With proper support, many people adjust beautifully to colostomies.

The diseases that are most likely to prevent effective reorganization are diseases that by their very nature cut the patient off from other people. Severe neurological diseases, massive strokes that wipe out speech and comprehension, syndromes that cause perceptual distortions, hallucinations, and memory loss—these are apt to be especially devastating since they attack not only the body, but the mind, which is at the very heart of our sense of humanness. Great sensitivity and patience are required of the physician who cares for such patients.

Occasionally, the symbolism of a disease to a person can critically affect his ability to adjust to it, as it did with Earl. Certain diseases strike particular dread in all of us: cancer, syphilis, leprosy, schizophrenia. Many patients are particularly fearful of contracting the illness that afflicted a parent. A man whose father died of a heart attack will spend his life fearing the event in himself; if it happens, he may be devastated even when his prognosis, from a physiological standpoint, is good.

The severity of illness is usually the least important factor in determining a patient's success or failure during the stage of reorganization. Usually, if one's mind is intact, a person can adjust to almost any physical reality, no matter how grave or disabling.

The Support System. The tolerance, understanding, and acceptance that an ill person receives from his family can be critical in determining the outcome of his reorganization.

I recently observed an interview conducted by a resident in Family Practice with a woman suffering from Crohn's disease. Over the years, her illness had pursued a downhill course. She had had many operations and now retained fewer than 3 feet of small bowel. The medical complications had been numerous. Yet, as I listened to her speak, and observed the animation and warmth in her face, it was clear that she was not depressed. She had retained, throughout her illness, a close loving tie to her husband and children. At one point, she described an incident in which her colostomy bag had exploded during a hunting trip in the Colorado Rockies. It was fall, but there was considerable snow on the ground. She talked about how she had had to take off all her clothes and, with her husband's help, wash herself off with handfulls of snow. Then, because she was cold and shivering and her own clothes were soiled, her husband had stripped down and given her a good two-thirds of his own clothes. She said to her interviewer with a laugh that she was sure they made "quite a pair." It was easy to admire their strength and tenderness. An incident that could have been, under different circumstances, messy, humiliating, and sad instead turned into a very special act of sharing and love.

Repeatedly, the relationship of a person to his family will be a critical predictor of outcome. Families that provide support can be of immeasurable value to us in our efforts to treat patients. Conversely, there are many unfortunate situations in which families abandon our patients or else severely sabotage their efforts at recovery, with catastrophic results.

The Effectiveness of Medical Treatment. Lorin Stephens, the clinician and medical educator quoted in Chapter 2, told this story about one of his own patients:

He had treated an elderly woman for many years for an arthritic condition. Over the span of their relationship, she had become very attached to him and trusted him implicitly. At a certain point in her illness, Dr. Stephens felt a knee operation would be necessary. She readily assented, and in due course, the operation was performed.

Then, while she was in the recovery room, a tragic error was realized. The wrong leg had been draped—Dr. Stephens had operated on the wrong knee.

After considerable anguish of his own, he did what he knew he had to. As soon as she had stabilized postoperatively, he told her the truth.

"Mrs. Fenswald," he began, "I have to tell you that we have made a terrible mistake. Through a series of blunders, I have to tell you that we operated on the wrong knee."

Mrs. Fenswald initially looked taken aback, then pensive. For a moment the two sat together in silence.

Then, Mrs. Fenswald replied. "You know, Dr. Stephens," she began, "I am obviously sorry that this happened. . . . But, I'm really not that worried. . . . You're such a good doctor, I'm quite sure the other knee will get better anyway."

It did.

Repeatedly, physicians will feel the power of something intangible yet unmistakable in the nature of the doctor-patient relationship that helps a sick person to get better. It is hard to overestimate the potency and curative potential of this very unique and special relationship. For all our technical advances, this relationship remains one of medicine's most powerful therapeutic tools.

And herein lies one of our most vexing problems. At the present time, our entire system of medical education emphasizes the content aspects of medicine—diagnosis, treatment, procedures—at the expense of the process side—the very human involvement of doctors with their patients. It is depressingly common to find physicians who are technological wizards, but interpersonal morons. They can treat disease but cannot seem to understand the person who has the disease. Such physicians are robbed not only of a potent therapeutic tool in their practice, but more fundamentally, they may be robbed of one of medicine's greatest pleasures, the opportunity to become close to another human being in a very special way at the height of life's most powerful dramas. Ironically, this is often the reason why physicians first enter medicine. Too often, it is forgotten. Medical education must change; it must begin to evolve in a direction that exalts the humanness of our work instead of ignoring it.

Often, as a teacher, I hear residents from different specialties complain about the drudgery of the outpatient clinic. Here, they say, is where the true "scut work" goes on, where the frustration is greatest. I hear laments such as, "At least when they're in the hospital there is something wrong—something you can do for them, something to treat." "These people here in the clinic. . . . " such residents will go on to say. "They have too many problems. Their lives are a mess. Their families are a mess. They just want to *talk*!"

Unfortunately, such residents have been taught to believe that the doctor's function is restricted to the management of acute disease. In contemporary medical practice, to an extent that was never true previously, doctors are taught to think of themselves as technicians who treat people only in stage two, the stage of Disorganization. They diagnose the ascites, they give the

Lasix, they lower the sodium. Then, the patient is discharged. Or else, to use the common parlance, they are given "a disposition."

Does this mean such people are disposed of? "Disposition" means nursing homes and convalescent centers; referrals for occupational therapy, physical therapy, social work, and occasionally psychotherapy. These "dispositions" are usually seen by doctors as afterthoughts—appendages attached to the patient's care, rather than central elements in it. Actually, the patient will be most engrossed in the stage of Reorganization during this period. It is here that a patient will either be able to pick up the pieces of his life or else become depressed and defeated. This has been known to physical therapists, as just one example, for years. Many physicians, trained to think of their role as involving only the stage of Disorganization, will fail to appreciate this. They are understandably perplexed, therefore, by clinic patients, chronic patients, and "people who just want to talk." One goal of this text is to emphasize the importance of the doctor to his patient during all stages of illness.

Our curing potential should be used to the maximum. We should treat people, not syndromes. In order to achieve this, we must begin to redefine what we do. We must begin to see that the medicine of our understanding, empathy, and compassion is just as important and must be administered with just as much care as the solutions we inject and the tablets we prescribe.

References

Allen, W. (Dir.): *Manhattan*, United Artists release of a Jack Rollins-Charles H. Joff Production, 1979.

Ashby, H. (Dir.): *Coming Home*, Hellman Enterprises Productions, 1978.

Becker, E.: *The Denial of Death*, The Free Press, New York, 1973.

Cassell, E. J.: Reactions to physical illness and hospitalization. In *Psychiatry in General Medical Practice*, edited by Gene Usdin and Jerry M. Lewis, McGraw Hill, New York, 1979.

Dickens, C.: *Great Expectations*, New American Library, New York, 1963.

Erikson, E.: *Childhood and Society*, W.W. Norton, New York, 1950.

Fitzgerald, E.: *Rubáiyát of Omar Kháyyám*, Grosset & Dunlap, Inc., New York, 1956.

Complete Grimm's Fairy Tales. Pantheon Books, New York, 1944.

Hitchcock, A. (Dir.): *Psycho*, Paramount Pictures, 1960.

Kübler-Ross, E.: *On Death and Dying*, Macmillan, New York, 1969.

Kulik, B. (Dir.): *Brian's Song*, Screen Gems, 1971.

Levinson, D. J.: *The Seasons of a Man's Life*, Ballantine Books, New York, 1978.

Lewis, S.: *Arrowsmith*, Grossett & Dunlap, Inc., New York, 1925.

Mahler, M. S., and Furer, M.: On the concepts of symbiosis and separation—individuation. In *On Human Symbiosis and the Vicissitudes of Individuation*. International Universities Press, New York, 1968.

Mann, T.: *The Magic Mountain*, Alfred A. Knopf, Inc., New York, 1927.

Pakula, A. J. (Dir.): *Klute*, Warner Bros, 1971.

Sheehy, G.: *Passages: Predictable Crises of Adult Life*, E.P. Dutton & Co., New York, 1976.

Solzhenitsyn, A. I.: *The Cancer Ward*, The Dial Press, Inc., New York, 1968.

Thomas, D.: *The Collected Poems of Dylan Thomas*, New Directions Books, Philadelphia, 1957.

Vaillant, G. E.: Theoretical hierarchy of adaptive ego mechanisms: A 30 year follow-up of 30 men selected for psychological health. *Arch. Gen. Psychiatry*, 24:107, 1971.

Young, T. (Dir.): *Wait Until Dark*, Warner Bros, 1967.

part II

THE INTERVIEW

chapter 5

BEFORE THE INTERVIEW

In medicine's folklore, special prominence is given to the significance of beginnings. The first cadaver, the first pelvic, the first death—everyone has a story to tell about these. The stories are sometimes humorous, usually biting, and often very poignant. Often they center around the student's "greenness," his underlying sense of inadequacy.

When Alan was a 2nd year medical student, he ended one of his first patient interviews by exhorting his patient, "If there's anything further you can do for me, please don't hesitate to let me know." Like Alan, most students approach their first interviews with anxiety about their own competence. Such anxiety is appropriate when one confronts important new clinical tasks. Paul's tense moments prior to meeting his patient in Chaper 1—his restlessness, "butterflies," and loss of appetite that morning—are common responses for students to have in these circumstances.

In our role as directors of a large interviewing course for freshman medical students at the University of Colorado, we often spend time at the hospital during the first few weeks to ensure that things are proceeding fairly smoothly. Even though we don't know every student by sight, they are easy to spot. Visibly anxious, they stand in small clusters waiting for their first encounters with patients, joking nervously with each other, peering intensely at the ongoing details of ward life that they do not yet feel part of. Their body habitus is tense, their expressions uneasy. Yet despite the obvious truth of the observations, it is useful to ask ourselves why? What is so inherently frightening about meeting a patient?

The answer is not simple, but at least three general issues seem to affect most students: (1) the student's self-consciousness about his role, (2) fears and fantasies about what constitutes professional behavior, and (3) uncertainty about how to proceed technically with patients.

THE STUDENT'S SELF-CONSCIOUSNESS ABOUT HIS ROLE

One outspoken but apprehensive student said to her preceptor: "You've brought a patient in here for us to examine. At least to talk to. You've implied that he's going to see a doctor. But the fact is, we're not doctors, and I think this is an exploitation. It's for us—it has nothing to do with the patient. Really," she half joked, "the patient would get about as much value from spending a half-hour with the gas station attendant across the street."

This is false, and her preceptor hastened to tell her as much. But it is how many students feel, at least some of the time. The beginning student, as he approaches his first patients, does not know how to regard himself. Is he an intruder? A learner? A data collector? A sympathetic listener? A detached "scientist" scrutinizing an object of interest? A friend? An impostor? Or is he the victim, along with his patient, of a contrived learning situation into which both student and patient alike have been forced?

The answer is all of these, at least to some extent—all, except a doctor. There is almost universal consensus on this among students: however else they may regard themselves, very few students view themselves early in their training as doctors, albeit beginning ones, with something unique and important to offer their first patients. Almost always, preceptors try to argue them out of this point, emphasizing that students are indeed physicians, though still in training, and will be seen by patients this way. Students in turn invariably react in one of two ways: either they feel the preceptor is trying to toss them a bone to make them feel better, or they suspect that he is encouraging them to be phony and to misrepresent themselves to their patients. In Chapter 1, Paul suspected Dr. Gellman of both.

The student in his first interviews is faced with a very difficult task. Limited in his knowledge of pathophysiology, he listens to patients describe signs, symptoms, and technical procedures, frequently with greater comprehension than he himself possesses. Even if he is only attempting to understand the patient as a person and to empathize in a general sense with how illness has affected his patient's life, the task is not easy. Interviewing a patient is no ordinary conversation and a great deal is going on. It can be quite difficult to listen on many levels at once—to listen to the emotional tone of what a patient is saying, to the content of his communications, to the process by which his remarks come up, to the mood in the room, and to a host of other subtleties that transpire during the interview. On top of this, the student typically is being watched by his preceptor, by his peers, and in a real sense by himself. It sounds almost glib, in such a situation, to assert that the best way to hear and perceive most in an interview is to be able to listen with a relaxed receptiveness! This is hardly a stance that one can expect a student to attain. During his initial interviews, the student is bound to feel somewhat uptight, which can't help but constrict his receptivity to some degree.

Beyond the complexity of the task to be performed, students also feel self-conscious. Typically, a student feels that he is on trial. The competitive system that got him into medical school and keeps him there obviously does little to allay these concerns. Even with the most encouraging and uncritical preceptor, however, many students turn out to be their own harshest critics—critics who watch vigilantly to see what kind of doctor this student will be, how patients respond to him, how good he looks in front of his peers.

Medical students throughout their training constantly find themselves in the unenviable position of being neither fish nor fowl. They barely get used to the routine of the basic science years when they are thrust into their clinical years. They have barely mastered those before they are "back to go" as interns. In the beginning years, when most introductory interviewing courses are taught, generally students are closer to identifying with patients than they are to thinking of themselves as physicians. Many of us have had the experience of being a patient. At the very least, we can readily imagine what it would be like. When students go up on the wards for their first interviews, they naturally feel helpless and out of place. They are foreigners in a milieu that seems to operate smoothly, incomprehensibly, and very much without them. The strangeness of a modern medical ward and the mysterious new technology that is everywhere conspire to make the student feel like an outsider in a foreign country. This enables most students to feel a very special sensitivity for bewildered and "lost" patients in this same situation. Such empathy can often contribute greatly to the unique relationship a medical student offers his patients, although he does not often value it highly. To begin with, he recognizes that he is not a patient. More important, he is trying to struggle his way out of the role of "complete novice" and to begin to see himself as a physician. Feelings of helplessness and bewilderment are seldom confortable. In his new role, as awkward and uncomfortable as a new white coat, the student finds himself already estranged from his earlier nonmedical identity yet not integrated into a new one. In this awkward hybrid state, the student must perform the difficult task of tyring to reach out and make contact with patients. It is clearly no wonder that students have a terrible time appearing "natural" with their first patients, much less feeling natural.

This inevitable self-consciousness in turn creates a kind of psychological "Heisenberg principle" in which the student's inevitable tendency to observe himself leads to a powerful interruption of his natural abilities to relate to people. Some of the old and comfortable ways of relating to people that he brings to training must in fact be given up and replaced by other skills as he begins to interact with patients as a physician. However, much of the native empathy and compassion for people that the student brings with him is valuable. When increasing self-consciousness alienates the student from his own empathic abilities, the experience can be unnerving.

At the outset of this chapter, we related the story of Alan's faux pas. In fact, Alan initially laughed with the rest of us when he realized what he had said. He later felt upset, however, for saying such "a stupid thing." He wondered what had happened to his old native talents in talking with people. It was particularly painful for him, because it was this very ease and pleasure in dealing with people that had led him to become a doctor in the first place. Now he felt that what once was spontaneous behavior had become an issue for endless dissection and technical consideration. Even such a simple matter as shaking hands at first meeting had become an object of concern. Should I shake the patient's hand? Do I shake hands with some patients and not with others? Should I stand by the patient's bed or pull up a chair?

A disruption similar to Alan's occurs at some point for most students. Not only do their natural mannerisms seem subject to excessive concern and scrutiny but also their basic perceptions and feelings. If the patient says something funny in the interview, is it all right to laugh? Or would that be "unprofessional"? The old intuitions about how to relate to people no longer serve as a guide, yet the new ones seem foreign, stilted, and often phony.

One of the central goals of an interviewing course, therefore, should be to help the student feel more at ease with patients and with himself as a beginning physician. Feeling at ease, however, is not the same as being jocular, social, or chatty. It involves the more difficult process of mastering heightened feelings of self-consciousness and moving gradually from a position of self-preoccupation to a more balanced involvement with the patient and the task of the interview.

FEARS AND FANTASIES ABOUT WHAT CONSTITUTES PROFESSIONAL BEHAVIOR

What is a doctor? Even in simpler times than these, people's perceptions of doctors were enigmatic, extreme, and often paradoxical. Is the doctor a wise, sympathetic healer who sits patiently at the bedside sometimes holding his dying patient's hand? Or is he the austere, emotionally unapproachable "brain surgeon" who nevertheless performs brilliant and miraculous operations? Images of the wise, humane physician commingle uneasily in our minds with the image of Dr. Frankenstein, the scientist who flirted with life's ultimate mysteries, who had commerce with forces dark and uncontrollable. In our current social climate, the paradoxes are even more abundant. The glowing accolades that accompany medicine's unparallelled technical advances coexist with an increasingly restive and suspicious public image of physicians as greedy, technologically obsessed, compassionless, incompetent, and grandiose. It is no doubt inevitable that anyone linked as closely with the fundamentals of human existence as a doctor would be perceived with such ambivalence. At no time in history have the paradoxes been more abundant and seemingly irreconcilable.

The physician himself is not immune to these fragmented and conflicting views of what a doctor really is. Doctors at all levels of training and experience are currently experiencing a considerable crisis of identity, self-esteem, and purpose. The beginning student is particularly vulnerable. In the midst of this confusion, the student has a strong and understandable psychological need for an image of stability, coherence, and confidence. Just as societies in times of great turmoil turn to strong charismatic leaders, so do students during a period of major internal upheaval and loss of identity search for some strong, charismatic image of the ideal physician.

The images, myths, and fantasies about this figure change over time for each student and vary considerably in their details from student to student. The common thread that links all students, however, is the wish for a model to aspire to and perhaps initially to imitate until its ideal characteristics can be internalized.

Three "caricatures" of the charismatic physician are identified below— there are doubtless more. They are the wise professor, the humane generalist, and Captain Medicine. Not only do these three images often commingle in a student's mind, but, more importantly, each figure is perceived with some ambivalence, as we shall see.

The Wise Professor

These are older clinicians, usually men, often department heads, almost always full professors. Often they wear long white coats and have at least some distinguished trace of gray. Typically they have achieved national prominence in some specialized area of research, but they also retain stature as senior clinicians.

Viewing them from afar, students see in such mentors symbols of absolute calm, inner equanimity, and unflappable self-assurance. These traits are most appealing at a time in the student's development when they hardly characterize his own experience.

On the other hand, students can perceive these same professors at other times in a very different, and negative way. They are the aloof administrators cut off from real patient care. They are the scientists, more interested in research than in human beings. Finally, like all patriarchal symbols, the wise professor walks perilously close to the "dottering old fool." It is not uncommon for a student's image of one of these heroes to be shattered when he hears younger housestaff say that this professor is, in fact, totally out of date and hasn't written "anything worth a damn" in the last 10 years.

The Compassionate Generalist

Call him Dr. Welby or Dr. Jones. For most medical students, as for much of society, there runs a deep respect and affection for our image of the wise, humane, warm family doctor. The recent resurgence of interest in family medicine among many medical students doubtless reflects this respect and perhaps a longing to get back to "the basics." As the popularity of the TV show makes clear, the basis of our longing for this archetypal hero runs deep. Take the lovely, famous poem by Robert Frost, "Stopping By Woods On A Snowy Evening," which we believe was written about a country doctor.

> Whose woods these are I think I know.
> His house is in the village though;
> He will not see me stopping here
> To watch his woods fill up with snow.

My little horse must think it queer
To stop without a farmhouse near
Between the woods and frozen lake
The darkest evening of the year.

He gives his harness bells a shake
To ask if there is some mistake.
The only other sound's the sweep
Of easy wind and downy flake.

The woods are lovely, dark and deep.
But I have promises to keep,
And miles to go before I sleep,
And miles to go before I sleep.

Certainly the poem is about much more than just a country doctor. Very possibly this briefly serene, solitary man symbolizes the artist himself midway in the journey of his own life. But it is also an apt symbol for the dedication, tolerance of fatigue, endless patience, and fundamental loneliness that we associate with the country doctor.

It is often the image of the compassionate generalist that most shapes a student's notion of physicianhood prior to beginning medical training. In most training centers, however, generalists are nowhere to be found. Thus, the image of the generalist's good qualities becomes based more on fantasy than actual exposure to real models. In contrast, students also hear a great deal that is pejorative.

The compassionate generalist is referred to by many housestaff as "the LMD" (local medical doctor)—a dumb jerk who is so out of date with recent journals that he can't order the right tests and sends his disasters to the medical center to be saved when it's all but too late. He is also a money grubber, an excessively affluent business man of medicine who owns two Cadillacs and a funmobile. Finally, he is an ignorant sentimentalist—a hand holder—because he lacks the skills and technical expertise to cure his patients of rare diseases. Many of these negative stereotypes are reinforced by the third charismatic type.

Captain Medicine

In our experience, it is the interns and residents who ultimately exert the most powerful influence as role models for medical students. This is less apparent in the first 2 years of medical education, when a great deal of time is taken up with basic science lectures. The clinical courses that are offered in these first 2 years—notably, introduction to clinical medicine courses—are typically taught by faculty. Early in the student's education, however, the image of the houseofficer emerges vividly. He is the exhausted yet somehow dashing figure toting a bellboy and dressed in surgical greens. He is the one who knows just what to do when that disastrous motorcycle accident is brought into the emergency room. He starts the i.v., gives the bicarb. He administers the cardiac massage. It is he who seems comfortable with the catastrophic, overwhelming, and unimaginable. It is he who has the latest journal article at his fingertips. Always, the student remembers that it is this figure who the student will become in just a few short years.

During the junior and senior years, resident housestaff exert a truly profound influence on medical students. Here is a description by one of the authors of his impression of houseofficers when he was a junior student.

> I remember those weeks vividly. The sounds and smells . . . I have never felt so helpless or inadequate . . . perhaps I was too impressionable. As I look back on the experience, it's clear I wasn't emulating the medical techniques of houseofficers, but rather their style of adaptation to stress. It was very strange. Under normal circumstances I would have seen these people for what they were: students a little older than I with strengths and weaknesses of their own. But somehow my sense of inadequacy at that time made it necessary to take them for models.
>
> Basically what I learned from my young mentors was that preparing oneself for an admitting night . . . is like preparing for battle. We don callousness like a suit of armor (DER).

Houseofficers epitomize both the best and worst of medicine. A seasoned 3rd year surgery resident may well be at the pinnacle of his emergency room prowess; his technical skills, his knowledge of the latest procedures, and his ability to implement them can be awesome. At the same time, he may be callous, brusque, and harsh to the people entrusted to his care. Overwhelmed by the demands placed on him—for omniscience in the face of sleeplessness, omnipotence in the face of overwhelming suffering—the houseofficer is not at a stage in his own development that permits him to be receptive to himself, warm, or well rounded.

Perhaps, partly from his own sense of guilt, this houseofficer is often prone to mock such qualities in other physicians. Generalists are handholders. Older clinicians are "behind the times." Medical students who show too much feeling for their patients are "impressionable" and "green."

Unfortunately, the feelings of many beleaguered houseofficers regarding patients and physicianhood may at times bear more resemblance to this poem by the contemporary poet, W.D. Snodgrass, than to Robert Frost's lovely couplets.

> Old Fritz, on this rotating bed
> For seven wasted months you lay
> Unfit to move, shrunken, gray,
> No good to yourself or anyone
> But to be babied - changed and bathed and fed.
> At long last, that's all done.
>
> Before each meal, twice every night,
> We set pads on your bedsores, shut
> Your catheter tube off, then brought
> The second canvas-and-black iron
> Bedframe and clamped you in between them, tight,
> Scared, so we could turn

You over. We washed you, covered you,
Cut up each bite of meat you ate;
We watched your lean jaws masticate
As ravenously your useless food
As thieves at hard labor in their chains chew
Or insects in the wood.

Such pious sacrifice to give
You all you could demand of pain:
Receive this haddock's body, slain
For you, old tyrant; take this blood
Of a tomato, shed that you might live.
You had that costly food.

You seem to be all finished, so
We'll plug your old recalcitrant anus
And tie up your discouraged penis
In a great, snow-white bow of gauze.
We wrap you, pin you, and cart you down below,
Below, below, because

Your credit has finally run out.
On our steel table, trussed and carved,
You'll find this world's hardworking, starved
Teeth working in your precious skin.
The earth turns, in the end, by turn about
And opens to take you in.

Seven months gone down the drain; thank God
That's through. Throw out the four-by-fours,
Swabsticks, the thick salve for bedsores,
Throw out the diaper pads and drug
Containers, pile the bedclothes in a wad,
And rinse the cider jug.

Half-filled with the last urine. Then
Empty out the cotton cans,
Autoclave the bowls and spit pans,
Unhook the pumps and all the red
Tubes—catheter, suction, oxygen;
Next, wash the empty bed.

All this Dark Age machinery
On which we had tormented you
To life. Last, we collect the few
Belongings: snapshots, some odd bills,
Your mail, and half a pack of Luckies we
Won't light you after meals.

Old man, these seven months you've lain
Determined—not that you would live—

Just to not die. No one would give
You one chance you could ever wake
From that first night, much less go well again,
Much less go home and make

Your living; how could you hope to find
A place for yourself in all creation?—
Pain was your only occupation.
And pain that should content and will
A man to give it up, served you to grind
Your clenched teeth, breathing, till

Your skin broke down, your calves went flat.
And your legs lost all sensation. Still,
You took enough morphine to kill
A strong man. Finally, nitrogen
Mustard: you could last two months after that;
It would kill you then.

Even then you wouldn't quit.
Old soldier, yet you must have known
Inside the animal had grown
Sick of the world, made up its mind
To stop. Your mind ground on its separate
Way, merciless and blind,

Into these last weeks when the breath
Would only come in fits and starts
That puffed out your sections like the parts
Of some enormous, damaged bug.
You waited, not for life, not for your death,
Just for the deadening drug

That made your life seem bearable.
You still whispered you would not die.
Yet in the nights I heard you cry
Like a whipped child; in fierce old age
You whimpered, tears stood on your gun-metal
Blue cheeks shaking with rage

And terror. So much pain would fill
Your room that when I left I'd pray
That if I came back the next day
I'd find you gone. You stayed for me—
Nailed to your own rapacious, stiff self-will.
You've shook loose, finally.

They'd say this was a worthwhile job
Unless they tried it. It is mad
To throw our good lives after bad;
Waste time, drugs, and our minds, while strong

Men starve. How many young men did we rob
To keep you hanging on?

I can't think we did you much good.
Well, when you died, none of us wept.
You killed for us, and so we kept
You, because we need to earn our pay.
No. We'd still have to help you try. We would
Have killed for you today.

Despite the pain expressed in this poem, students are usually quickly surprised to discover how therapeutic their interactions with patients turn out to be. Usually students quickly rediscover the strength of their own personalities. Positive patient responses and appropriate reinforcement by the preceptor lead to a reawakening of confidence in the student's own natural abilities. It is a vulnerable period, however. Like a seedling, the student's re-emerging self-esteem needs a fertile climate of support, meaningful encouragement, and helpful criticism to grow. A few put-downs or an upsetting or disruptive patient interview can leave the student feeling unsure again. Unfortunately, we all too often witness the phenomenon of students who begin to develop a sense of themselves, only later to feel humiliated by more advanced students and houseofficers.

It is important to remember that, in a world increasingly populated by technologists and machines, the most precious gift a doctor has to offer a patient is still himself. Rediscovering the therapeutic potential of one's own personality, therefore, is one of the important goals of any introductory interviewing experience.

UNCERTAINTY ABOUT HOW TO PROCEED
TECHNICALLY WITH PATIENTS

The most immediate concerns students have prior to beginning an interview are pragmatic. How do I introduce myself? What if the patient says he doesn't want to be interviewed? What happens if I don't understand his disease? What happens if I say something to upset him and make him feel worse? What happens if he has a cardiac arrest and drops dead in the middle of the interview? The questions seem endless. In fact, the issue of how to begin with patients is as fundamental as how to think of oneself as a physician. How does one approach the patient in a physicianly way? How does one convey his sense of competence? No interview outline, however well considered and inclusive, can accomplish this. There simply is no armamentarium of sure-fire techniques that the student can bring with him. It is impossible to be fully prepared for the fluid, unpredictable process of any physician-patient interaction.

In some ways, the best advice prior to any interview is, "Just go and do it." Yet such advice does not seem to convey empathy when it is offered, and students generally feel frustration when preceptors keep reminding them of how stressful and ambiguous the process is. Students want answers! Surely something can be written down in black and white that is more precise than generalities about one's emerging identity, changing role experiences, and the like. Students may well appreciate that there is no foolproof map to lead them through the thicket of questions and technical considerations that arise. At the same time, the wish for some concrete guidance is reasonable. In this section, therefore, we will address a number of beginning issues that students commonly face.

Introductions

The question of how to introduce oneself to the patient immediately raises a knotty issue—should I say I'm a doctor? Current educational trends suggest that the student be completely honest. But what is being "completely honest?"

"Good morning, Mrs. Smith, I'm Mark Brown, a medical student—a freshman medical student. This is only my first month of school and this is an introductory course. I really don't know much about medicine but they told me I should come here and interview you to ask you how you feel about your illness and all—ah, that is, if it's all right with you?"

While this seems a bit exaggerated in print, it is, in fact, typical of the way students tend to introduce themselves. Why? Are such lengthy disclaimers really for the patient's benefit? In our view, medical students often have a greater need to disclose their novice status than is necessary for the patient's understanding or comfort. They may do this to protect themselves. It is as though the student is issuing a disclaimer: "I'm not really a doctor so don't expect anything from me." This reduces the student's anxiety, but is it, in fact, truthful? Do patients really perceive medical students as being little different "from the gas station attendant across the street"?

The answer is, no. For most patients, the exact nature of the medical hierarchy, and different people's status in it, is never entirely clear. This may not be ideal, but it tends to be a fact. With the exception of certain chronic patients who have had complex ongoing care in teaching hospitals, most patients have little grasp of the difference between an intern and a junior student much less between a junior student and a freshman. As uncomfortable as this may feel, most patients regard medical students as doctors. They confer on the student both the prestige and responsibility that the title Doctor demands.

We recommend, therefore, that introductions be brief: it is sufficient to identify oneself as a medical student and then to give a brief statement of the purpose of the interview. If the purpose is to talk about the patient's response to his illness in general terms, then say so. If the intended scope of the interview is broader, including the obtaining of a medical history, it is sufficient to say, "Good morning Mr. Smith. I'm Mark Brown, a medical student, and I'd like to spend some time talking with you about the troubles you've been having." Such an introduction is sufficiently general to permit the patient to begin where he wishes—either with the specifics of the medical history or with different concerns. The doctor later has plenty of time to focus in on more specific concerns.

Many students feel a need to include some statement that the interview is taking place as part of a course. This is often defended in the name of honesty, yet it is open to question. Sometimes students do, in fact, obtain important information about the patient that becomes a part of his record and may influence his management. Furthermore, telling the patient that the interview is for a course may be one more way the student has of minimizing the prestige and responsibility that he is endowed with. Still, if students wish, it is perfectly acceptable to say that the interview is part of a course.

The question of introductions raises another controversial issue. It is the current trend for students to introduce themselves as Mr., Ms., or Mrs. Interestingly, 10 years ago the trend was quite different and students were encouraged from the beginning to call themselves doctors. Has this change come about to protect the patient from deception? Is it a reflection of our greater enlightenment and humility? Perhaps. But we would at least like to raise the question of whether calling oneself Mr. or Ms. isn't potentially as misleading to a patient as calling oneself "Doctor." In legal terms, a medical student presumably becomes a doctor on a given day in June when he graduates. Or does he? Is it rather when he receives his state license? After internship? After completion of housestaff training? Even legally, the issue is not clearcut. Ethically, it is even more cloudy. Most physicians train for a minimum of 8 years. At what point along the continuum are they doctors? Obviously, the answer is—at all points. The limits a student places on his interventions and responsibilities should depend more on his own grasp of his limitations and capabilities than on an official title. A junior student alone on a ward will conduct a cardiac arrest until more help arrives, if he must. Is he not a doctor? On the other hand, a 2nd year medical resident may wisely defer to a more experienced houseofficer in performing a tricky liver biopsy. Is he any less a doctor? If, then, patients tend to regard students as doctors; if, in fact, the student assumes a responsibility the minute he introduces himself to the patient—to listen, to attempt to understand, perhaps to contribute to the information on the patient's chart—which then is really more misleading, to call oneself Mr. or doctor? We raise the issue not to encourage deception. We know full well that most students prefer to begin calling themselves doctors after receiving their M.D. degree, usually at the beginning of an internship. This is reasonable enough. We have dissected the question at some length because this seemingly simple content issue— like so many others in medicine— is far more complicated when one takes a deeper look.

The White Coat

We recommend that students wear white coats during their patient interviews. We recognize that this is not the prevailing trend at many medical centers, where "appropriate dress" is the rule of thumb but not specified. Nevertheless, we consider the white coat a reassuring symbol of physicianhood for the patient. As in the matter of calling oneself "Doctor," some students argue that wearing a white coat is deceptive. To the contrary, we feel that *not* wearing one is an act of denial and is inconsiderate to the patient.

Consider the patient's vulnerability. He may be told that he is going to be interviewed by a medical student, "a young doctor," or "a student physician." However it is defined, 9 times out of 10, the patient anticipates an interview with "a young doctor." He expects to disclose feelings and intimate details about himself that are private and personal and may leave him feeling vulnerable. Yet, patients are generally willing to do this because they are speaking to a doctor. In this sense, we feel that donning a white coat is a symbolic act of commitment—an expression of the student's willingness to be responsible to the trust the patient places in him.

Despite this logic, some students may still choose not to wear a white coat. Sensible standards of dress should then be a minimal requirement. For men, this means a clean, pressed pair of slacks, shirt, and tie; for women, a dress, a skirt and blouse, or a comfortable yet not excessively casual pair of slacks and blouse or sweater. Again, however, we recommend the white coat; though it has fallen out of popularity, it remains a potent symbol of physicianhood to most patients. The use of a nametag is also strongly recommended.

Confidentiality

In a busy medical center, it is common to overhear clusters of doctors inappropriately discussing their patients in public places. Often the details they discuss are intimate, specifically identifying, and quite frightening to the visitors and nonmedical personnel who crowd into the elevators and cafeteria lines with them. How this loss of consideration has become so widespread raises some disturbing questions about the way most medical centers are run. It goes without saying that patient confidentiality is an absolute expectation for anyone treating patients but most especially for physicians—including student physicians.

In many ways, the importance of a commitment to confidentiality is internal. In reality, a casual reference to some patient, spoken too loudly in the elevator, is apt to be forgotten by whoever overhears. But, the student's commitment to honor his patients' communications as a sacred trust—this attitude is directly related to an emerging sense of oneself as a doctor.

Students sometimes have questions about where to draw the line. Talking among peers is appropriate in one setting, yet not in another. Furthermore, should the student go home in the evening and discuss the matter with his or her spouse? One could answer this rigidly with a resounding, no! Never! But the truth is, almost every student (and, for that matter, every physician) at some point discusses a case with his or her spouse. It is doubtless wrong to do so. Yet we physicians sometimes strap ourselves with Draconian standards of perfection that are hard to fulfill. A student may well go home at night feeling exhausted yet quite overstimulated. The spouse may be the only person to turn to and share with. Similarly, it is often very difficult for the nonmedical half of a relationship to be left in the dark about the exciting and intense activities that comprise the medical student's days. Therefore, there are no absolutes. However, a good rule of thumb is: no patient should ever be identified by name, and any discussion of patient contacts with close friends or spouses should be general and focus more on the student's side of the experience than on anything specific about the patient.

Finally, it is well known that doctors frequently group together and joke about patients. In the safety of a back room, they laugh about someone, call him names, make wisecracks. It is easy to condemn such behavior; yet one must understand the plight of the physician. Overwhelmed and overloaded he can sometimes find relief in comraderie through humor, even sarcastic humor. It can provide a useful release that then enables the physician to return to work and behave in a humane and professional way with a difficult patient. Yet students should also be aware that jokes, casual or cruel jargon, and slang can quickly lead to a mind set in which physicians begin to think of patients as "crocks," "turkeys," and "gomers." If doctors think of patients that way, they are bound to treat patients that way, and if they do treat them that way, they are bound to get a response in kind; and thus the vicious cycle is completed.

Confidentiality and the highest level of respect for the patient's dignity are therefore worthy aspirations. Although we all fall short of this goal at one point or another, we should try to discover the underlying frustration that motivates such humor. Perhaps in finding an answer to this question we may find a way more effective than mockery to cope with a difficult patient.

Closeness

Many students wonder about the appropriate distance to set with a patient. Usually patients tend to set the distance themselves, though some patients tend toward one or the other extreme. Some, for example, stand excessively aloof. Others become excessively regressed, demanding, and clinging. Students likewise have different degrees of tolerance for closeness. A bit of "chemistry" goes into this. Some students, for instance, can tolerate angry, hostile patients better than seductive ones, while others find their undoing in excessively dependent, clinging patients, and so forth.

Generally, the experienced clinician develops a capacity for empathy that permits fluid shifts between closeness and detachment. At different times during an interview, an experienced interviewer can be almost at one with the patient emotionally, identifying with his pain and inner suffering, then shifting quickly into detachment and objectivity—sliding back and forth along an axis of closeness-distance as the situation warrants. This is far more difficult for the beginner. Typically, early in clinical exposures, students find themselves vacillating between overidentification with patients and excessive aloofness and detachment. One student referred to this as "not knowing how to regulate my empath-o-stat." In fact, the problem of establishing a balance may be another important motivation for the laughter and gallows humor that we hear among physicians. It is possible that caustic, barbed humor is a way physicians have of mitigating the excessively tender feelings that patients may arouse.

The concrete questions that students raise about closeness are many: Should I sit on the patient's bed? Should I hold his hand if he cries? What if the patient asks me to hug her? As much as he would like specific guidelines, the student will probably appreciate that there really can be none. In general, professional contact should be conducted primarily through words. A great deal of empathy and concern can be communicated to most patients through language alone. Occasionally, holding a patient's hand or a reassuring touch are both necessary and appropriate. The student should be cautious, however, because body contact is a potent intervention that often has significant, though sometimes unconscious, meaning to a patient. This is an area that takes time to master and one in which the understanding of an experienced preceptor can be especially helpful.

Another specific question that many students have centers around self-disclosure. Patients can, and frequently do, ask students questions about themselves. These can range from the quite chatty to the very intimate. How and when does a student respond to these questions, if ever? Again, there are no absolute rules. Some students seem to try to caricature the physician as a pseudo-Freudian statue who stonewalls every personal question. Obviously, this is rude and unempathic. At the other extreme, some students seem ready to answer every question that a patient asks, from the state of their marriage to the age and health of their parents, without ever asking why the patient seems to want to know all these things. A general principle (alas, not a rule) is that less self-disclosure is preferable to excessive self-disclosure. The doctor-patient relationship is one in which the doctor must be essentially unselfish and focus primarily on the patient. Sometimes this must be said to a patient so he will understand.

Similarly, students may find themselves having strong feelings about patients. Some patients evoke great feelings of tenderness, admiration, protectiveness. Others may evoke frank feelings of contempt and revulsion. Sometimes students wonder whether to share these feelings with patients. We will talk more about the use of such feelings under our discussion of countertransference in Chapter 7. Generally, however, it is unwise to tell patients directly how one feels about them. There are usually more tactful, therapeutic ways of transmitting the same information. Take, for instance, the highly demanding, interrogative patient who keeps asking detail after detail regarding the medical student's exact level of expertise and training. The student may feel, "I'm getting increasingly annoyed with this man's attack on my credentials, on my right to be here interviewing him." To say so directly might well be honest, but not especially helpful to the patient. Recognizing the feeling, however, the student could well say, "You seem to be concerned, Mr. Jones, about whether or not I will be able at my level of training and expertise to understand you. In fact, it sounds to me like you're worried about whether the entire staff is up to the task of helping you as much as you need and deserve." In both interventions, an awareness of an intense feeling leads to a response to the patient. But in the second response, the intervention is shaped in a way that does not specifically disclose the student's angry feelings toward the patient nor needlessly put the patient on the defensive.

Age

"But doctor you look so young!" These words can be the student's nemesis. Actually this expression is a common manifestation of many different kinds of patient concerns. From some patients, the remark is unquestionably a put-down. Other patients may be expressing real apprehensions about the competence of someone who "looks so young." In some elderly patients, it can actually be an expression of delight. The student may remind such patients of a beloved grandson or granddaughter.

Unfortunately, the question tends to do wonders toward making egos wither. If the student can withstand the implied insult, however, it is often very helpful to then explore with the patient in a congenial way what the student's youth means to him.

It is usually not necessary for the student to tell a patient his exact age, though patients will occasionally insist. It is far more productive to ask oneself, "Why is the patient asking me this question? What underlying concern is he expressing?"

Concerns about youthfulness also lead to concerns in two related areas: invading a patient's privacy and interrupting.

Invading a Patient's Privacy

Many students are concerned about the right they have to pry into the intimate details of a patient's life. It is always interesting to observe the student who will practice some procedure on a patient, such as inserting an i.v., without questioning his right to do so, yet who will then protest vigorously against obtaining a sexual history because it constitutes using the patient as a "guinea pig for my learning."

Reluctance to pry becomes more pronounced when the patient is elderly, when the problem is sexual, and when there is a gender difference between the student and patient.

Delving into a delicate matter obviously requires tact and a willingness to back off. Yet, usually patients are very anxious to talk to a professional about these very matters, which often concern them greatly. Usually it is the student who cuts these patients off, from his own sense of discomfort. A receptive silence will often bring forth tears from patients, but along with them will come intimate disclosures about sexual concerns, body changes, grief, and depression. Allowing this to occur, and recognizing it as therapeutic, can be difficult for many physicians. Yet, in our culture, many patients turn to the physician as the only one who is willing and able to listen. In the busy, congested milieu of a hospital ward or clinic, it is often only the student who offers these patients the opportunity they need to open up. In Chapter 1, Mrs. Clark opened up a great deal to Paul. Yet, how much more might she have opened up, had Paul been more comfortable still about having her do so? About any men in her life? About her sexuality? We know these issues were on her mind from her discussions about her appearance, her need for a wig, and her assertion that she had once been attractive. How much further might she have been willing to reveal herself about these matters, had Paul indicated a willingness to listen?

Interrupting

Many students fear interrupting a patient. This is especially prominent when the patient is elderly.

During our interviewing class at the University of Colorado, we ask many older patients to volunteer for a videotape interview with the students. These patients are almost always enthusiastic about working with medical students and excited about the contribution they can make. They willingly come to the University to be interviewed about very real health problems they have and are eager to talk to someone about how they are adjusting to their illnesses. During the videotapes these patients generally talk enthusiastically, volubly, and often nonstop about their lives. With few exceptions, however, the interviews all look remarkably the same—the patient smiling cheerfully, talking on and on, with the student sitting, hands folded in lap politely smiling and nodding but rarely interrupting.

When the students are asked afterwards how they feel about these interviews, the majority complain that they have been hard to conduct. They feel in conflict about whether or not to interrupt their elders. They are afraid of appearing rude and insensitive. As one student put it, "I felt like I needed to raise my hand for permission to speak before I asked a question."

Fear of a Patient's Crying

A group of students was interviewing a patient with chronic and disabling arthritis. During the course of the interview the patient sighed several times and spoke with much sadness about being confined to her home as she became more crippled. Her story was depressing. At one point, she quietly began to cry. Shortly before the end of the interview, one of the students stepped up to her bedside and began a casual banter, telling her jokes, asking her about some of her favorite card strategies and how she had developed an interest in bridge.

In the discussion that followed among the students and their preceptor after the interview, the students all agreed that the patient had told a depressing story. The student who had engaged the patient in social banter stated that he had become afraid in the interview that the patient would lose control and start to cry. He feared that the effect of their interview would be to make the patient worse. He therefore felt a responsibility to comfort her by cheering her up.

The ability to deal with a patient's crying is a difficult skill to master. We go into medicine to relieve suffering, not to cause pain. Yet experience soon tells us that we must constantly hurt patients—with needles, knives, and catheters; sometimes with the truth; and sometimes simply with a receptive silence and a willingness to stick with the emotions that the patient brings up, for these evoke a flood of feelings. The therapeutic value of permitting a patient to express pent-up, painful feelings is hard to overestimate. Yet many students and many patients fear that if a patient starts to cry he won't be able to stop. This rarely happens, of course, and no one has ever died of tears. Often it is enough in such situations for the student to offer the patient a tissue, perhaps to touch the patient's hand, but above all to show in his expression and manner a sense of concern. Usually, the student should remain quiet, communicating to the patient in this way that it is all right to cry, or get angry, or express fear.

Here again, the student has a unique therapeutic potential. Chances are, in most training institutions, he will be one of the few with the time and patience to allow his patient to open up in these ways. As for the therapeutic importance of this, one can certainly think of Paul's interaction with Mrs. Clark in Chapter 1 as a clear example.

APPROACHING THE FIRST INTERVIEWS

Much of the above has centered on what could be called rules of procedure—dress, protocol, and appropriate physicianly behavior. Beyond these rules, there are a number of inner assets and external allies that the student brings with him to his patient interviews.

A Sense of Purpose

If a student enters an interview with a negative mind set—that he is exploiting the patient, using him as a guinea pig for his course, etc.—it is obvious that he is not going to feel a sense of purpose. If, on the other hand, he approaches the interview with a recognition of his potential contribution, then a clear sense of purpose can be conveyed. The student's potential contribution includes an opportunity to review important information from the medical history (perhaps uncovering new information), a chance to give a human being in distress emotional and psychological support, and finally an opportunity to permit the patient to open up about serious concerns that he may not have been able to express before.

As stated earlier, introductions are important. Whether the student's purpose is restricted to understanding the patient's illness in a general sense or also includes formal history taking the student can invite the patient to speak about "what brought you to the hospital" or "what sort of troubles you've been having."

In the more general beginning interview, organizing questions include: How does the patient feel about his illness? What effect has the illness had on his life? On his job performance? On his capacity for social and physical activity? On his family? A simple, rather than technically exquisite and detailed, discussion of symptoms is appropriate. When did the symptoms begin? What changes did the patient notice? How did the symptoms progress? Keeping these questions in mind can give a general sense of the interview's purpose. The student can ask himself, as the interview proceeds, whether there are pertinent issues remaining to be explored in these areas. Thus, these questions can serve as guidelines without unduly restricting the interaction. Checklists, standard questions asked over and over with different patients, are generally ill-advised, as they usually fail to elicit the most important information and tend to put the patient off.

The student may also be able to clarify for the patient certain aspects of how his treatment is proceeding—the type of treatment offered, the rationale for the medical regimen that he is receiving, the various members and functions that comprise his health care team. Obviously, the student will sometimes have to say "I don't know." At the very least, however, students can be helpful in assisting a patient to articulate what his areas of confusion are, what questions he needs to ask, and of whom he should ask them.

Finally, if the scope of the interview includes obtaining a history of medical illness, past history, and review of systems, the purpose and organization of the interview become much more precise. This will be discussed in Part III. The student should beware, however, of a tendency on the part of physicians to become excessively preoccupied with the strictly somatic aspects of the patient's care to the exclusion of a concern for his emotions. We have seen many physicians who literally cannot approach their patients comfortably unless they are holding up a stethoscope or other piece of medical equipment in front of them. Frequently, as students become more adept at obtaining a content directed medical history, they forget more and more to focus on the patient as a person. One can see how tempting this is. Talking to a patient about what is really going on with him emotionally can often be painful, depressing, and a little frightening. Yet, enabling the patient to talk about these matters is an essential part of the patient's overall therapy. In this area, the beginning interviewer may actually have an advantage; knowing less pathophysiology, he may have fewer verbal smokescreens to hide behind. This may enable him to get closer to the patient than a more experienced clinician often does.

Thinking of the Patient in Developmental Terms

A number of recent authors, both in scientific publications and in popular literature, have stressed that human beings go through stages of the life cycle, "passages," throughout their adult life. We all continue to grow and change throughout our lives. Yet, until recently, the stages we pass through have not been fully elucidated; most studies of psychological development seem to stop at adolescence, or even earlier. An excellent book about the developmental stages of adult life is Gail Sheehy's *Passages*. Reading this book can assist the student to refine his curiosity about patients at different stages of life. A young accountant in his 30s who develops a heart condition, for instance, will have very different concerns than an elderly man in his late 70s with the same medical problem.

Whether or not the student actually reads further in this area, however, it is useful to organize one's curiosity around the developmental stage of the patient. If a patient is 50, what does the student imagine are some of his concerns? Aging? The growing reality of eventual death? Children leaving home? If a student knows how old his patient is, in other words, it is well worth thinking about what issues the patient must be facing in his life. This sense of curiosity can provide the student with another source of perspective and structure in the interview.

Empathizing With the Patient's Anxieties

As nervous as a student may be before his initial interviews, chances are the patient is also quite nervous. Imagine for a moment that you are a patient in a busy teaching hospital. There is another patient in a bed close to yours. You told the head nurse who came in an hour ago that you would consent to be interviewed by a medical student. What do you expect? Probably you envision a young person, dressed in a white coat, somewhat formal, "doctorly" in presentation and manner, serious and earnest. You might expect that person to look intelligent. And you would probably assume that the student will talk to you in much the manner that your other physicians have. You might rehearse the history of your symptoms—when they first began, where the pain was first located, at what point you went to the doctor. You know that these are questions doctors ask. But perhaps you will also worry about the impression you make. Will you discuss your symptoms intelligently and coherently? Or will this student, like the doctor you saw 2 days ago, get impatient with you for rambling on about "unnecessary" details? And how do you look? You've not had a chance to shampoo. Will the student notice the sack of urine hanging down at the foot of your bed? Will the smell from your infection bother him?

If the student is able to imagine himself lying in bed waiting to be interviewed, his empathy for the patient's beginning anxieties will be enhanced. This can also give clues to issues that may be on the patient's mind at the beginning of meeting. Even though talking about his medical problem may be the stated agenda, the patient is also going to be concerned about the impression he makes on you, just as you are worried about the impression you will make on him.

A 40-year-old woman was being interviewed postoperatively, following an evacuation for a subdural hematoma. At the beginning of the interview, she seemed highly agitated, fidgeting with her hands, allowing her eyes to dart about the room, tugging at the buttons on her pajamas. At first, the student wondered to himself what he had done wrong—how he was making such a bad impression. He then began to wonder, however, what the patient's anxieties were. At this point, he simply observed that she looked a bit anxious. "I look awful!" she blurted out. The nurses *promised* me they'd give me a chance to wash up and put on my make-up before you came to interview me!"

Attentiveness to Affect

Often interviews seem fragmented, disjointed, and difficult to follow. Themes emerge, then disappear. One minute the patient is talking about her gallbladder. The next she is discussing her fifth cousin in Omaha. It is understandably difficult, therefore, for the beginning interviewer to know initially how to follow the different threads. A useful organizing principle is to follow the affect. In general, every interview will have an emotional tone, which may range at different times from anxiety, to humor, to elation, to depression and boredom. While the content of a patient's communication may often seem opaque, if a student tunes into the underlying emotional tone of the interview, a much greater coherence often becomes apparent.

A 60-year-old woman with congestive heart failure was talking to a student about her illness, especially her frustration at not being able to walk as far as she once had. She greatly enjoyed her recreation. In passing, she mentioned that she and her husband had both been avid bird watchers prior to his death 2 years previously and she missed getting the exercise. Soon, she began to ramble. There followed expressions of sadness—she would heave great sighs, look out the window, turn her eyes away from the interviewer and fidget with a magazine. The student did not know quite what had happened. At the time the interview was breaking down, the patient was talking about nothing in particular, actually about the dosage of her Digitalis. The student had not yet learned the concept of process (which we will discuss in Chap. 6), but he did know the patient looked sad. "You seem sad to me," he said. At this point, tears welled up in her eyes and she said, "I still miss him so. It's been 2 years but I still think about him every night and cry myself to sleep. He was a good man!" Thus, even though the student did not know why the patient was sad, knowing that she *was* sad was sufficient to organize and refocus the interview.

Paying attention to the emotional tone of an interview can be one of the single, most reliable organizers that the interviewer has. In this regard, attention to process is central to understanding what transpires during patient interviews. This concept will be discussed in detail in Chapter 6.

The Preceptor and Fellow Students

The preceptor can do a great deal to set the stage for a student's beginning interviews. Having seen a demonstration interview, for example, many students have commented that a great deal of benefit accrues to hearing the cadence of a well conducted interview by an experienced interviewer. The preceptor may assist in introducing the patient to the student, either at the bedside or in the clinic setting. He can clarify for both patient and student the broad nature and purposes of the interview that will take place. In addition, part of the preceptor's function may include some introduction of the student to the facility itself, its workings and the individuals comprising it.

We recommend that students do their interviews in the presence of their preceptor and peers. Although their presence can augment the sense of self-consciousness that we discussed earlier in the chapter, as an interview proceeds, the preceptor and fellow students are in a unique position to observe and later comment and advise. They can follow many themes and nuances of an interview that emerge that inevitably escape the attention of the interviewer because of his absorption with the patient. Thus, their presence provides a double benefit. The observers have the advantage of seeing the interview unfold at a more relaxed distance. The interviewer himself has an equally unique and valuable set of impressions forged in the more intense crucible of his direct engagement with the patient. The preceptor's ability to monitor the general process of the interview, to rearticulate it coherently and comprehensibly, can be invaluable. Likewise, feedback from fellow students about what went on during an interview, which interventions of the interviewer did or did not work, can also be extremely helpful in enabling the student to develop increasing mastery of his interviewing style.

The preceptor and student's peers can serve another very important function. It lies in the empathy, support, and understanding they can offer to the student conducting the interview. In discussions after the patient interview, students sometimes feel that preceptors are treating them with kid gloves, not giving them enough substantive critical feedback. To an extent, this is probably true. While preceptors' approaches vary greatly, those who are skilled at teaching interviewing recognize that a student's specific technical mistakes are less important than his developing sense of professional style. Thus, in well run groups, the student often feels a great sense of support, understanding, and empathy. The importance of this is not simply to provide an experience in which the preceptor and peers are "nice." Specifically, as the preceptor and fellow students empathize with the student's thinking and feeling during his own experience, the student actually experiences what feeling another's empathy is like. It is through this process, perhaps more vividly than any other, that the student comes to appreciate the therapeutic power of accurate understanding and empathy in the doctor-patient relationship.

The Student

It would be incomplete to close a chapter on assets that the student brings to his patient interactions without speaking of the student himself. It is always sad to see students over the years of their training increase in technical proficiency and content knowledge yet seemingly lose faith in the therapeutic value of their own personalities. Unfortunately, our medical education system often reinforces this.

From the outset, students bring many skills to patient interviews. One of these is the skill of observation. This skill is initially untrained. As it becomes more developed and refined, it becomes one of the major skills a physician possesses. Ask yourself what you observe about the patient when you walk into his room. How was he sitting in the bed? Was there a magazine on his lap? What was its title? What article was it open to? Was the patient on the phone? What did he say before he hung up? How did he first greet the student? What was his color? Did he seem to move with pain when he shifted posture? What was the color of his fingernails? What was the first remark he made?

Often in the rehashes that follow an interview, students are amazed when their preceptors remember these details and point them out. Often a single observation seems to cast a whole new light on the meaning of the interview. Students often wonder how they will ever become so observant. Yet, if one examines the phenomenon closely, students usually *do* recall having observed these things. Usually there is a sudden response of recognition and the student says, "Yes, I remember that—now that you remind me!" Thus the power of observation is not lacking but rather the power to make these observations accessible to one's conscious awareness. This ability comes with time. It requires the gradual development of an ability to pay attention to an interview on several levels at once—the patient's words, mannerisms, appearance, moods, all at the same time.

Another important native talent that most students bring to their interviews is curiosity, about bodies and the way they work, about minds and the way they work, and about how mind and body work together or against each other. In one sense, much of good medical interviewing consists of curiosity. A natural curiosity leads to appropriate questions and, in fact, it contributes greatly to the phenomenon of clinical intuition—the hunch— that is so important at all levels of experience in medicine.

In a real sense, all students are experienced interviewers. They have spent a lifetime listening to people and attempting to understand them. Generally, they have sensed in themselves a special interest and sensitivity for other people that has led them to choose medicine as a career. It is true that students have a great deal to learn as they transmute a native interest in people into internalized, reliable ways of dealing with them as professionals. Nevertheless, it would be a great mistake to depreciate the knowledge and experience that the student already brings with him. Each student has his own personality and style. Furthermore, no matter how much a student learns, his style will remain the fundamental basis of his interactions with patients throughout his professional lifetime. This is why techniques alone cannot create a skilled interviewer. The skills to be acquired do include specific techniques but they can never encompass the real task for the beginning interviewer, which is to get in touch with who he is himself and with what it feels like to be a patient, and then to develop those insights into a coherent professional style.

Finally, the student brings to his interviews something else that is very special—a sense of responsibility. While this is not restricted to physicians, we feel that a sense of responsibility and deep commitment to another human being is one of the essential hallmarks of physicianhood. By the very fact of his presence in medical school, and his presence—however awkward and nervous—before a patient, the student is making an important statement: "I am willing to listen to you and to try to understand you. If I can, I will try to help you, but above all, I am committing myself to be responsible for you."

A desire to comfort a patient, to make a deep ethical commitment to him—this is one of the basic qualities that distinguish a good physician. "To cure occasionally, to help often, to comfort always" is the motto engraved over the Hotel Dieu in Paris, an early forerunner of the modern hospital. This ancient motto expresses a very human notion that should not be forgotten by the student as his content knowledge increases and his technical skills advance.

References

Frost, R.: Stopping by woods on a snowy evening. In *A Pocket Book of Robert Frost's Poems*, Washington Square Press, New York, 1946.

Lipkin, M.: *The Care of Patients: Concepts and Tactics*, Oxford University Press, New York, 1974.

Reiser, D. E.: Struggling to stay human in medicine: One student's reflections on becoming a doctor. The New Physician, *22:*295, 1973.

Sheehy, G.: *Passages: Predictable Crises of Adult Life.* E. P. Dutton & Co., Inc., New York, 1976.

Snodgrass, W. D.: "A Flat One." In *After Experience*, Harper and Row, New York, 1960.

chapter 6

THE INTERVIEW PROCESS

A black physician was interviewing a white patient. The patient was coopera-
tively if somewhat distantly relating his medical history. The patient then interrupted his history reporting to ask the physician if he had seen last Sunday's
football game. He told the physician admiringly how impressed he was with an
80-yard run by O.J. Simpson. The physician, sensitive to the process level of his
patient's communication, responded that O.J. Simpson was indeed one of the
nation's foremost black athletes. The patient nodded. The physician then asked,
"Have you ever been treated by a black physician before?" This sensitive interchange greatly facilitated the patient's being able to discuss his particular concerns
about this particular doctor, and increasingly *with* this particular doctor.

A central concept to the understanding of any interview is the concept of
PROCESS. An understanding of the process of an interview will enable the
student to understand central and critical themes being communicated by
the patient in that interview. For example, an understanding of process
communication enabled the physician in this vignette to grasp the subtly
stated concern of his patient; he was thus able to open this area to discussion
and so to foster the development of greater rapport. The physician here
responded to the process level of his patient's communication by asking
himself why the patient chose to tell a casual anecdote about O.J. Simpson
in the middle of the medical history; he realized then that the patient's
mention of a black athlete might have something to do with how the patient
felt about being treated by a black physician. Learning to identify, understand, and use process in this way is initially challenging. But its rewards are
substantial for both patient and doctor.

There is a process level in all communication between people. It is not a
concept restricted to doctor-patient interactions. In every interchange, people
talk and listen; but as they do so, an endless series of silent questions,
associations, and thoughts run through their minds. Imagine, for example,
that you are at a cocktail party. Imagine specifically that you are standing

with an interesting but unfamiliar stranger. You are curious, so you begin to make small talk. You talk about sports or the weather. You ask each other about your interests. This is the surface of your interchange. But it is quite obvious that something else is unfolding between the two of you, below the surface. Behind the small talk, you are actively sizing each other up, in some ways of which you are aware, and, very possibly, in others of which you are not. What is going on between you at this level is *process.* You may be silently asking yourself, "Is this person intelligent? Warm? Is he (she) a good listener? What does he (she) think of me?" In such a social situation, at a cocktail party, you are not apt to pay too much attention to the process level of your communication, though it is there. You are there to socialize and have some fun. To ferret below the surface for "deeper meanings" in every human interchange would be amateur psychologizing and really wouldn't be much fun.

One can understand, however, that when doctor meets patient, the process level of communication between them becomes extremely important. So much of what is important to a patient when he is sick will be communicated in process. A person who falls ill feels anxious, depressed, angry, and frightened and has a host of other feelings that accompany illness. Often, however, the patient is not aware of these feelings explicitly, and just as often he is unable to express them to his doctor directly—at least in their initial meetings. The patient can communicate these concerns only at the process level. This is why it is so important for a physician to understand how to tune in to these communications. For instance, the vignette with which we began this chapter illustrates a concern that is almost universal in patients: "Can this doctor take care of me? Can I trust myself to be in his hands? Will he understand me?" Sometimes patients are aware of such concerns, sometimes not; but they almost never bring them up directly. They do, however, communicate them in process, as this patient did.

RECOGNIZING PROCESS

Students usually find that once they begin to develop a facility in understanding process, interviews become more alive; the patient and physician emerge as unique and exciting individuals. One patient is not like the last. One doctor is not like the last. One of the real pleasures of understanding process is that the nice surprises that are so much a part of the human interaction between doctor and patient begin to unfold. They occur continuously, from small, isolated seemingly inconsequential interchanges to the sum total of the interaction from start to finish.

How then does the student begin to recognize and work with process? Although it takes time and experience to get good at it, a student can begin to understand the process level of his patient's communications if he constantly asks himself three essential questions during the interview: (1) Why is the patient telling me this *now*? (2) What is the patient telling me about his *feelings now*? (3) What is the patient telling me about his feelings regarding the relationship between *him and me now*?

1. Why is the patient telling me this *now*? "Why now?" may be the single most important question a physician asks. A patient contracts pneumonia. The critical question is, *why now*? A patient develops a new complication in the chronic course of his diabetes. Why now? The central importance of this question in a patient's medical history will be discussed further in Part III. Here, it is sufficient to say that this question is the single greatest clue to what a patient is communicating on the process level. Why did the patient come *today* for treatment? Why has the patient come to the emergency room *tonight*, complaining of headaches when headaches have been a chronic problem for which the patient has not sought treatment for years. Why, as the patient talks, does he choose to make a specific comment or bring up a particular question now?

One patient in the hospital for a routine hernia operation interrupted the doctor's history taking to ask about the seriousness of his frequent headaches, which he had had for years. The doctor talking to this patient asked himself why the patient brought up this question, seemingly out of context, now? He then found out, upon inquiry, that the patient was worried because his father had died 5 years earlier from a brain tumor. By asking himself "why now" this physician was able to tune in to important concerns in his patient that the patient was communicating on the process level.

Though the patient was really in the hospital only for a minor surgical procedure, thoughts of death were very much on his mind—memories of his father's death, fears that he too would die in the hospital as his father had. Similarly, in the vignette that began this chapter, it was the physician's ability to ask himself, "Why does the patient talk about O.J. Simpson *now*?" that enabled him to understand the concerns his patient was having in the doctor-patient relationship.

2. What is the patient telling me about his feelings *now*? It is obvious that patients have very strong feelings when they are ill. There is good evidence, both in folklore and more recently in the scientific literature, that strong feelings can cause illness, even death. The doctor's awareness of his patient's feelings can have a tremendous influence on the patient's clinical course in ways that range from trust and compliance to the speed with which a patient recovers. It is entirely appropriate for physicians to be especially concerned with the factual details of a patient's illness. If a patient comes in with chest pain, the physician must find out about his symptoms in depth so that he can make an appropriate diagnosis and develop a treatment plan. But the data he gathers are only as reliable as the atmosphere of rapport, empathy, and trust in which he gathers them. It is important to remember that, no matter how critical the "hard data" may be to the physician, patients are invariably consumed with concerns of an emotional nature. They want to know whether they've had a heart attack. Will they live? Will they need an operation? Can this doctor take care of me? She looks so young. He looks so old. Although such concerns will vary from patient to patient, they will most often be communicated to the physician on a process level. Therefore, it is important to underscore the need to ask the question, What *is* the patient feeling, *right now*?

3. What is the patient telling me about his feelings regarding the relationship *between him and me now*? When a patient comes to a doctor for treatment, he comes with a problem—physical, psychological, social, whatever. As soon as he begins to interact with the doctor, however, something important invariably occurs. Quickly, his feelings about his relationship with that doctor become at least as important to him as the problem that brought him in for treatment. These concerns are almost always expressed by the patient at a process level.

It is no exaggeration to say that during an initial interview between a new doctor and patient, almost all of the patient's communications *on one level* will relate to how the patient is feeling, *then and there*, about placing himself in the hands of his doctor.

The vignette with which we began this chapter illustrates this clearly. So do many important interactions between Paul and Mrs. Clark, described in Chapter 1. Think back to the episode when Paul did not wear his white coat, and Mrs. Clark began to talk about her older brother, Sam—how Sam experienced responsibility thrust upon him, whether he felt ready or not. This is a common way for patients to communicate in process, through displacement, and we will explicate it further below. But even without an explicit understanding of process, Paul sensed (somewhat to his discomfort) that what Mrs. Clark was talking about through displacement—a seemingly random anecdote about an older brother—actually had a lot to do with her relationship with Paul.

This concept tends to make some doctors quite uneasy. Most doctors are initially skeptical about the notion that so much of what a patient is saying under the surface has to do with his feelings about the doctor. One obvious reason for the discomfort is the awareness of responsibility this realization fosters. If a patient is talking, on a process level, so much of the time about how he feels about his doctor, that puts quite a bit of responsibility on the doctor's shoulders. This is, in part, what made Paul feel so uncomfortable with Mrs. Clark.

Another reason for physicians' skepticism is their feeling that it is somehow vain, conceited, and egocentric to think that so much of what a patient is saying has to do with the doctor himself. No one likes to see himself as self-centered. Yet, with increasing experience, the clinician will repeatedly have this point brought home to him: whatever problem might have brought the patient in, once the interaction between them begins, how the patient feels about the doctor is of paramount importance in the patient's mind and is constantly being communicated on a process level.

THE VARIETY OF PROCESS TRACKS

Process communications have a rhythm, timing, and sequence of their own. Important communications occur simultaneously on multiple levels. To begin to recognize them, an analogy is useful. Consider the comparison with modern studio recording techniques. A musician may begin by recording one "track" on a tape, for instance, the melody line or the lyrics. He will then add other tracks—the bass line, the piano, other parts of the orchestra. By the time the musician has finished, he may have recorded as many as 16 tracks that are coordinated to produce the final piece of music. In an analogous manner, process communications can be seen as simultaneous tracks. Of these, the surface content—the factual, concrete words that the patient is saying—form one track only.

Below we have enumerated 12 common "process tracks." Their numerical sequence does not imply that any one track is at a greater "depth" than any other in the patient's mind. Nor is this list exhaustive. The important thing to keep in mind is that all of these tracks play simultaneously as the patient and doctor communicate.

1. Process communications occasionally—though rarely—speak plainly and openly in words. Once in a while, a student encounters a patient who tells him directly how he feels during the interview. Usually this is more common in experienced patients who either have had chronic medical treatment or else have had many experiences in teaching hospitals. For example, one obese 65-year-old female patient told her student physician very directly, "You can ask me any questions you want, but don't draw no blood from me. I have hard veins and I've been stuck too many times by inexperienced doctors like you." There's no mistaking how the patient is feeling here. Even in this instance, however, it is possible that there is further process hidden beneath her seemingly forthright expressions of distrust. For example, it turned out that this particular patient often "attacked" new doctors as a way of keeping distance and not running the risk of future disappointment.

In any case, patients usually do not express their innermost concerns so directly.

2. Process communications speak about the present by talking about the past.

> A 45-year-old man with chronic active hepatitis was talking to a female medical student. Spontaneously, he told her about how his wife had left him 10 years previously—how hurt he had been, how hard it was to cope after she had gone. With some help from her preceptor, the student was able to formulate the question "Why is the patient telling me this *now*?" She realized then that he was talking about his relationship with *her*. She had gotten to know this patient over several interviews during a 16-week course in the doctor-patient relationship. Just a few minutes before, she had told the patient that her duties there would be ending and she would not be seeing him anymore. The patient was telling her, in process, how sad and disrupted he felt that he was losing her as his doctor.

Talking about the past as a way of communicating feelings and concerns n the present is an extremely common way for patients to express their oncerns in process.

3. Process communications are often expressed in displacement.

> A 60-year-old physician's wife was in the hospital to begin renal dialysis for advancing kidney failure. A medical student was interviewing her for the first time. To his frustration, she refused to talk about her illness, going on and on

instead about her avid interest in trout fishing. She talked about a big one she had caught and mounted a few weeks back. She described in detail how disappointed she was when the fish was finally mounted. "In the water it was so sparkling, and fresh and alive," she said. "By the time they skinned it and stuffed it and pounded it on to a board all of its beauty was gone." After the interview was completed, the student shared this material in his preceptor group. As they discussed it, they began to realize that the patient's discussion about the fish was in fact a displaced way of talking about herself. She was afraid that as her kidneys failed and she became more dependent on machines to keep her alive that she, too, would lose her vitality and luster and "aliveness."

Patients frequently speak in displacement as a way of expressing concerns that they're having *right now* in the present.

4. Process communications hide their most important messages behind "trivial" passing remarks, "by the ways," and casual "jokes."

A 56-year-old married businessman, hospitalized for a suspected myocardial infarction, was talking to a medical student. Although he was obviously afraid for his future, he would only talk about this in the most roundabout way. He chatted amiably about his business and his plans for expanding it "after I recover." Finally he asked her, "What about exercise, doctor?" The medical student said, "I *think* it will be okay after you recover but probably you should take that up with your doctor, Dr. Jones." The patient agreed that that would be a good idea. "Maybe I will," he said. Then, pausing, he commented, "So you're a medical student, huh? How do you like it?" He went on to ask if she had taken anatomy yet. The medical student responded factually that she had. The patient made a face. "Ugh!" he exclaimed, "That part would upset me. It would be hard. Seeing all those dead bodies. I admire you kids." These remarks were made casually, almost as a chatty aside, toward the end of the interview. When the student asked herself why the patient brought this issue up *now*, however, she realized that the patient had just previously been talking about his concerns for the future and his chances of recovery. It then became clear that on the process level this patient was saying to the student that he was afraid he was going to die and end up as a corpse in the morgue.

5. Process communications make their point by linking together emotional themes.

A 45-year-old construction worker was in the hospital with advanced kidney disease. Due to his illness, he had lost a great deal of weight. His wife was present while a medical student interviewed him and told the student that her husband had valued his once strong, robust physique and fretted about all the weight he'd lost. The patient himself, however, would say nothing about this. Instead he launched into a rambling discourse that sounded to the student like nothing more than a gripe session. In a gruff, "macho" tone of voice he complained about the jerks down at the job who were holding up his disability payments. He complained about his oldest daughter who was "nothing but a hippie" who only came home when she wanted to take something from him, like money. One of the nurses on the night shift was giving him a hard time and wouldn't give him his sleeping pills when he asked for them, but he was going to take the matter to the hospital administration. "All the way to the top if I have to!" He was going to get redress for all the wrongs that had been inflicted on him.

In the group discussion that followed the interview, the students were initially perplexed by the meaning of this patient's complaining. The preceptor suggested that they might look for any common themes in his complaints. After some discussion, the students all agreed that two themes were very important. First, the patient was complaining about being cheated and robbed. Second, he was asserting in no uncertain terms that he was nobody's fool and would get his due. It then became much clearer to the students what those *themes* might have to do with how the patient was feeling about being very sick with kidney failure *right now*. They decided that his complaints about being "robbed" probably grew out of his anger—he was upset that his illness had "robbed" him of his health and vitality. As for his assertion that he would get back at anybody who stood in his way, the students concluded that he way trying to reassure himself that he was not weak and helpless; he was showing the world that he was still a strong, capable man who could look out for himself.

6. Process communications speak through body language. Recently, the whole subject of body language has received considerable attention in both medical and lay publications. Serious medical books try to explicate the way a person "speaks" through his body. Lay publications promise to teach the reader how to read somebody's innermost thoughts, fears, and conflicts. The latter claim may be somewhat exaggerated, but body language *is* a very important avenue through which patients express themselves. The patient who says to the doctor, "How nice to meet you," but does not get up from a reclining position in her bed and extends a cold sweaty hand, is telling the doctor something very different from the patient who sits up, leans forward, and reaches out to shake hands upon greeting the doctor, even though both patients may use the same words. Body language at the beginning of an interview is particularly revealing. A student who can observe a patient when he first walks into the room to interview him, noting the position the patient assumes, the way he sits in the chair or bed, the degree of eye contact, can learn a great deal about how this patient is feeling about meeting his new doctor.

Some students tend to focus heavily on body language in their first encounters with patients as an avenue to understanding process. There is nothing wrong with this; the concept is exciting and innovative. The messages in a patient's posture and physical manner are reliable and relatively straight forward, once we become aware of them. Most students know innately what one posture is saying as opposed to another, once they consciously tune in to them. Furthermore, it is quite reasonable for a student in his initial interviews to rely on the straightforward guideposts that body language frequently provides. As a student becomes more advanced, however, he usually begins to integrate his understanding of body language with many other tracks through which patients communicate their concerns in process.

7. Process communications speak through a patient's shift away from a topic. The patient with a suspected myocardial infarction, who was described in track 4 above, exemplifies the importance of noticing how patients shift *away* from what is concerning them the most. Here is a part of the dialogue that transpired between the medical student and her patient:

> Patient: It's not that this one attack is the end of the world—if I take it as a warning. Stop smoking. Learn to relax more. Cut back a little at the job. It's important to do those things, isn't it, doctor? I mean, if people do change their lifestyle I've heard it's possible to go for years, maybe even forever without another heart attack. What about exercise, doctor?

At this point, the student recommended that he discuss this with the medical resident taking care of him. The patient responded: "Hm, that's a good idea. Maybe I will . . . so you're a medical student? How do you like it? My son—he's 18—wants to be a doctor. Is this part of your training?" Clearly, the patient, in this instance, shifted away from his concerns about his health to seemingly innocuous "chit chat" about the medical student's training and career plans (though, as you recall, the "chit chat" soon wound up on the subject of corpses in morgues!).

Students express themselves in process by shifting away from subjects as much as patients do. This interchange is a good example. When the patient asked advice regarding exercise, the medical student made a special point of saying that she didn't know, since she was only the medical student. She encouraged the patient to ask his resident, implying that he was "the real doctor." By shifting away from the patient's request for information here, the student too was communicating something in process. She was saying to this patient, in essence, "Deep down I'm not sure I feel like I want to be in charge yet. This level of responsibility makes me uncomfortable. Therefore, I will remind you at this point that I am not your real doctor."

8. Process speaks through shifts toward a topic.

A 55-year-old businessman, hospitalized with rectal bleeding from a diverticulum in his colon, was being interviewed for the first time by a medical student. Clearly, these two were not "birds of a feather." The businessman was conservative in his political views with strong convictions about the importance of fighting communism. His student interviewer had flowing blond hair tied back in a ponytail and a neat but bushy beard. The patient interrupted his discussion of the onset of his symptom of rectal bleeding to ask the student how he felt about gun control. "First, the liberals will try to take our guns," he asserted. "Then, the next thing you know they'll start chiselling away at our constitutional rights." He then asked the student if he didn't agree.

This student, adept at understanding process, asked himself why the patient had shifted to this topic now. He decided that the patient was feeling him out about their obvious differences—that the patient was probably expressing, in process, his anxieties about placing himself in the hands of a doctor who had views that were probably so different from his. The student said, "You're wondering about my political views. Maybe you're wondering, if I look at the world differently from you, whether that will mean that I won't be able to understand you as a doctor and take adequate care of you." Although the patient shrugged this off, in words at least, he subsequently relaxed and began to open up and trust more. There was little doubt that the student here had understood the process level of the patient's communications and, as a result, the rapport between them quickly grew.

9. **Process communications speak by evoking emotional reactions in the doctor.** Understanding process also includes understanding subtle feelings that a patient arouses in us as we interview them. Why do we find ourselves getting bored, tired, irritated, or sad? Inexperienced clinicians often feel guilty or uncomfortable about having such responses to their patients; but in fact these provide invaluable—often subtle—clues that enable one to understand what the patient is expressing on a process level.

The medical student who interviewed the physician's wife in renal failure, described in track no. 3 above, found himself getting bored. During the interview, the woman talked endlessly about trout fishing and the virtues of back country travel in Wyoming, while the student found himself looking out the window of her hospital room, imagining how nice it would be to be riding his bicycle home. He wondered what his wife was cooking that night for dinner.

In the discussion that followed the interview, the student was initially reluctant to confess these feelings. He felt somehow to blame for getting so bored and distracted. His preceptor suggested a notion that seemed somewhat radical but also worth pursuing: "Assume," his preceptor said, "that what you are feeling was evoked by the patient, and tells you something about the patient. What do you come up with?"

The student, after some thought, said that his boredom had, in effect, shut the patient out. It was as though she didn't matter. When he tried to think how his patient could have *made* him react in this way, he came up with an interesting notion: was it possible that this was because the patient's behavior toward him was saying that *he* didn't count? She was clearly a woman used to being in control, and she was having trouble adjusting to being a patient. Her way of coping was to denigrate, in a variety of ways, the student's importance to her. His boredom—which said in effect, "This patient doesn't count"—was a response to the patient's communication to him, that *he* didn't count.

Some students find it difficult to accept the idea that their feelings toward a patient may be due more to the patient's behavior than to some problem that they are having. Students are often reluctant to "blame everything on the patient," and doubtless a student's reactions sometimes have more to do with the student than with anything going on in the patient. Generally, however, if an encounter with a patient elicits strong emotions from the student, especially if they are uncharacteristic for him, it is wise to ask: "Could this patient be communicating something to me, however subtly, that is causing me to have these feelings?"

10. **Process repeats itself when it is not "heard."** Many students worry

that they will miss the most important elements of a patient's concerns if they aren't immediately adept at reading communications on the process level. One of the remarkable, and very reassuring, facts of medical practice, however, is that our patients give us many chances; patients communicate what bothers them many times and in many ways. There is no danger of missing any one golden opportunity. In fact, it is the *repetitiveness* of a patient's concern in some area that often alerts an interviewer to its importance to the patient.

> A 58-year-old brick mason was being worked up on the admitting unit of a university hospital for a possible myocardial infarction. Periodically, he interrupted the flow of the medical history to ask his doctor what he could do about "being tired all the time." His doctor was, of course, much more concerned about his chest pain at that point in time. However, in the coming days the patient kept asking in a variety of ways, "What makes middle-aged men get tired? What can be done about middle-aged fatigue?" After this patient's immediate medical problem had stabilized, the intern asked more about his fatigue. It turned out that the patient was really using fatigue to express his anxieties about some recent problems with sexual impotence.

Certainly the first order of business in this patient's management was to treat him for a possible myocardial infarction. Later in the hospitalization, however, the intern was able to help his patient get appropriate counselling regarding his sexual concerns, which were obviously of great import to him as he referred to them repeatedly during the interview.

11. Process communications are often expressed "outside" the interview. Patients have a remarkable propensity for saving their most important communications for those moments when they think it's "off the record." For example, they often make very telling remarks before the interview officially begins. One 68-year-old woman "joked" to the instructor who was introducing a medical student to her before the interview, "Who in the world would want to interview an old ding-bat like me?" It turned out that she had recently been put in a nursing home, after having lived for several years with her son and daughter-in-law. Issues of low self-esteem, and a feeling of being unloved by others, were expressed very poignantly in this little "joke" that preceded the interview.

Similarly, students who pay attention to what happens "after" the interview will be fascinated by the frequency with which important process communications occur. It is a very rare patient who does not continue saying *something* after the student has said, "It's time for us to stop now." Many patients begin to chatter at this point or ask a thousand more questions. Often they are saying, in process, that the student has meant something important to them and they don't want to let him go. Sometimes, they express their innermost fears only in these endings, "off the record."

> A 50-year-old truck driver with cardiac problems secondary to high blood pressure had chatted affably and, it seemed to his student interviewer, very superficially throughout their interview. After they had closed the interview and

shaken hands, the patient called out to the student when he was already half-way through the door. "Hey doc," he called out. "There is one thing I wanted to ask you. Who does a person call around here if they want to donate their bodies to the medical school?" The student returned to follow this patient up a day later and, of course, found that this patient had many concerns about dying.

12. Process communications often take the form of questions and requests for information. Patients frequently ask a variety of questions regarding medical students' level of training, their age, their experience, etc. Because students are self-conscious about this themselves, they are usually inclined to take such questions at face value. There is, of course, nothing wrong with giving straightforward answers to these questions. If a patient wants to know if you are a freshman, and you are, say so. But beyond answering patients' questions, students should also ask themselves, "Why is this patient *asking* this question?" The patient in track no. 9 above, who began asking his student doctor about his political beliefs, was also *telling* the student something very important about his underlying concerns. Patients rarely ask questions that are not also important statements of what is on their minds. Sometimes the meaning is obvious, as with the patient who asked his interviewer about donating his body to science. Sometimes the meaning can be more subtle.

One patient, a 45-year-old man with pancreatitis, asked his student interviewer, "Do they do any hernia operations here?" The student replied factually that they did. When he asked the patient why, it came out that the patient's oldest brother had died totally unexpectedly 5 years previously from complications after a routine hernia operation, performed in another hospital.

Another patient, admitted to the hospital for elective back surgery, seemed fascinated by the workings of the hospital lab. Over and over he would ask the student questions about the lab. Where did they store the blood? How many tests did they run a day? How many machines did the hospital own? The student tried to answer as many of the questions as he could, but was perplexed as to why his patient found this subject so fascinating. It came out later that the patient had recently seen a movie about hospitals. In it, he had been horrified that a number of patients had died when they were given the wrong medicines and operations in a series of terrible mix-ups. Once the student found this out, he was in a much better position to help this patient discuss his underlying concerns about his upcoming operation.

These 12 process tracks in no way represent an exhaustive list of the modes through which patients communicate in process. They are simply some of the more common ones. Some patients tend to express themselves more in one mode than another. Once a student begins to get a sense of how process language operates, however, he will know it when he hears it, even if the mode is quite unique. One patient kept her doctor informed of what was on her mind every day by telling him the latest developments in her favorite soap operas! This rather creative way of communicating was unique to her and certainly wouldn't be found in any standard text! Also, the student who is beginning to think in terms of process should not worry about memorizing this or any other list. The single most important guide is always the question: "Why is the patient telling me this now?"

A DEMONSTRATION OF PROCESS

In the next part of this chapter, we will present the transcript of an interview between a 1st-year medical student and his patient, a 70-year-old divorced white woman with arthritis. We will use this example to present the basic technical components of an interview—the phrasing of questions and such elements of the interview as transition, facilitation, empathy, and closings. Throughout, we will discuss the process communications that are occurring.

During this interview, the student clearly learns a great deal about his patient in a brief time. Prior to the encounter, the student was instructed to conduct a 15-minute interview focusing on the effect of illness on the patient; therefore, the medical data he gathers are not complete. Nevertheless the picture that he develops of this patient is extensive and contains critical information about her which, when it is later combined with complete medical data, will be important for her future care.

The patient appears to be an active woman who uses many gestures and expressions in the initial segment of the interview, more so when she is discussing certain areas.

THE INTERVIEW

S: Hello
P: Hello. You're my doctor, huh.
S: Yes. I just came from the other room. My name is Bill Green. (Student extends hand and sits down.)
P: Nice to meet you.
S: And yours?
P: Martha Walters.
S: Martha Walters?
P: Ah huh.
S: How are you? Where are you from?
P: Oregon.
S: You're from Oregon.
P: Well, originally from the East, and then Oregon, and for 2 years, Colorado.
S: Ah huh. So you're living here now.
P: Yes.
S: I see. And what brought you here? Why did they pick you to come over here (to the medical school to be interviewed)?
P: Well, I have a history of arthritis (putting hand to neck to rub it).
S: Ah huh.
P: You could start with that 'cause that's what hurts the most.
S: I see. And do you understand basically what we are doing—that we're freshmen and we're sort of . . . you know, obviously we're not interested in the illness . . . I don't understand it completely . . . but more generally the effect it's had on you.

P: Well, yes. All right. Um. (Pauses, wiggles in chair, covers eyes with hands.) I never feel that the arthritis stops me very much except it slows me down terribly in the morning and on cold days like this . . . it's in my neck (pointing to neck).

S: I see.

P: So, it's very, very, very sore in the morning. It's real agony.

S: How old are you?

P: 70.

S: And when did it start? How long have you had it?

P: About 3 years ago.

S: Three years ago?

P: I've had arthritis a long time. I started in my late 30s with arthritis but ah . . . you know I didn't believe it (laughing and shifting in chair). (*Author's note*: The laughter and body language here indicate that this is a painful area for the patient. Perhaps she *still* doesn't want to believe it.)

S: Your 30s, really?

P: Yes.

S: And this was all in your neck area?

P: No, no, it was in my hands, in the joints (lifts hands to inspect them).

S: In your hands?

P: There is some in my hip and I noticed that the doctor told me some time ago that I had a limp . . . without my noticing it . . . that I was favoring the hip (rubs hip). That doesn't bother me . . . just once in a while.

Introduction

An introduction should establish the interviewer's name and other pertinent identification, i.e., medical student, preceptor, and the plans for the interview. The patient's name should be asked and/or clarified. (Introductions are also discussed in Chap. 5.)

Questions

Simple Question

A concise question expressing one thought, i.e., How old are you?

Open-ended Question

A question that lets the patient answer in his (her) own terms; i.e., Why did they pick you to come over here?

Directive Question

A question that seeks to clarify or validate previous information; i.e., And this was all in your neck area? In general, it is better *not* to ask compound questions—questions requiring more than one answer at once. Bill did this when he asked, "How old are you? Where are you from?" Usually, this will cause the patient to answer only one of the two questions. The other question becomes forgotten by both patient and interviewer and important information may be lost. This is precisely what happened in this interview, though Bill does remember to ask Mrs. Walters her age again later.

Analysis of the Interview Opening

Beginning an interview can be difficult. Opening the avenues of conversation and setting the proper tempo can be challenging tasks for the experienced, as well as beginning, clinician. The task becomes easier with experience, as organized systems of inquiry develop. But whenever two people who do not know each other first meet, there will be a certain halting and awkward quality to their interaction, as is evident in this beginning.

In this first segment of the interview, Bill begins to develop, if somewhat haltingly, some identifying information with Mrs. Walters about her place of residence. This "thumbnail sketch" initially serves two important functions. First, information about age, marital status, place of residence, and occupation is important background that will provide diagnostic information as the patient's medical evaluation proceeds. This point will be discussed further in Part III. Second, obtaining identifying information initially provides a gradual and appropriate transition into the interview, allowing time for both patient and student to get their bearings.

Perhaps somewhat abruptly, Bill shifts his focus from this introductory phase to the medical problem. "Why did they pick you to come over here?" Also, on the process level, his saying "Why did *they* pick you ... " may suggest that he does not feel as if he really is in charge. Mrs. Walters identifies her problem as arthritis and then something interesting happens. Twice, when she says "it hurts," Bill goes back to the identifying data:

P: *You could start with that 'cause that's what hurts the most.*
S: *I see. And do you understand basically what we are doing—that we're freshmen.* (p. 122)

P: *So, it's very, very, very sore in the morning. It's real agony.*
S: *How old are you?* (p. 123)

Here the process of the interview is communicated by a shift *away* from an important topic. Bill shifts from "it hurts" back to what may feel to him like emotionally safer ground: "I'm only a student." From "it's real agony" to "how old are you?" Clearly, his patient's expressions of pain are uncomfortable for him. He signals that discomfort by shifting *away* from these concerns to a more neutral subject.

Watch what happens to the questions in the next segment.

S: Now this was when you were 30? That you actually noticed it?
P: Late 30s. About 39. 38 or 39. I can't really remember but about then, and the hands gradually got worse but, ah, they didn't stop me. (Lifts hands to inspect them, works fingers.)
S: It looks like you can work them pretty well. (Student mimics patient, working his fingers.)
P: Yea, I mean, I never stopped working them and I think this hurts me more than anything recently, and this started just recently (pausing to inspect hands and work fingers). Disgusting, my hands are a mess today because I've been working in my files.
S: So, what do you do? You said files.

The patient is communicating an important message here in the process. This is an example of a process communication that takes the form of a *seemingly* casual "aside." "Disgusting, my hands are a mess today . . ." she says. The patient is telling Bill something important. Here she is, being videotaped for an unknown "audience" and meeting a new doctor. She tells him, in process, that she's worried that her illness—symbolized by her deformed hands—has made her "disgusting," not just today, but all the time. Bill doesn't pick up on this here, for he responds to the literal content of what she is saying: "You said files." One could speculate about what Mrs. Walters might have said had Bill said something like, "You use the word 'disgusting.' Do you sometimes feel bad about your hands?"

P: Oh, no, that's just my own special stuff—it's something I do at home. I don't work . . . is that what you mean? (Squirms in chair, shifting positions back and forth, rubbing hands as though cold.)

S: Okay, but what have you . . . have you worked since you were 30?

P: No, I never had to work. Once in a while I would get a job if I was . . . when I first went to Oregon, when we did, I was bored and I got a job in a library. Most of my school training was music. Classical music and then library . . . a little bit of library work, so I've always been familiar with the library and that's what I do here. I volunteer . . . over at . . . with the books.

S: Are you married?

P: I'm divorced. (Patient repetitively socks palm of one hand with fist of the other, like a prize fighter.) (*Author's note:* The body language speaks for itself here.)

S: You're divorced? So you were married while you were developing this, but . . .

P: I've only been divorced a couple of years.

S: I see. Do you play an instrument? (*Author's note:* Here is another instance where Bill signals his discomfort by shifting *away* to a "safer" subject.)

P: I play the piano.

S: You do! (Student's tone is one of surprise and pleasure.) (*Author's note:* Some students think that to be "professional" means being somber and neutral. Bill's spontaneous expression of warmth here is most appropriate and bound to build rapport.)

P: Still do.

S: You still are able to do that?

P: Type all the time.

S: And you type?

P: Hm Hm . . . lately those two fingers aren't doing their job (works index and middle finger). I mean on the typewriter.

S: Can't reach out far enough?

P: Well, I can reach out but they've lost their strength (moving fingers in deliberate typing motion), so I'm hitting wrong letters. So I tell whoever I'm writing to if you don't like that, ignore it (laughing).

Here again, the process communication takes the form of a laughing "aside." "If you don't like that, ignore it." This is also an example of a process communication through displacement. The patient is supposedly talking about friends, people far removed from her and Bill. She is saying, with a bit of a stiff upper lip, that she worries that her illness will alienate people and turn them off. But then, with a bit of bravado, if they don't like it, they can lump it. She is also saying something in this displacement about her relationship to Bill. She is saying, in process, "I wonder what *you* think of me. Do I turn *you* off?" Then, through her bravado, she asserts that she wouldn't *really* care. But, of course, she does care!

> S: Does that cause any problems with your teaching at all?
> P: Teaching? I don't teach.
> S: You don't give lessons?
> P: No. No. I had a very fine musical education and I just always played 'cause I liked to, that's all. I have a big piano. And ah . . .
> S: So what about the neck problem? (Student rubs his neck.) Has that been debilitating at all to you? Has it . . . other than just in the mornings. Does it go away?

Transition

A transition is a specific and planned attempt to change the topic, to leave one area and move to a new one. The object of transition is to provide continuity and structure during the interview. The transition here leaves something to be desired. Students frequently feel awkward moving from one subject to the next. Some are not sure when to leave an area or how. As mentioned in Chapter 5, some students are reluctant initially to "take charge." A statement here such as, "Your music sounds like a real delight for you; but for now I would like to return to talking more about your arthritis. Is arthritis debilitating for you?" provides a smooth, tactful, and understandable break and redirects the conversation.

> P: Well, I've always said, no, and I think it isn't debilitating. It started to be last summer, but I had a couple weeks in the hospital and over at the arthritis clinic hospital—I always call it the arthritis clinic.
> S: Where is this?
> P: I'm trying to think of it. Memorial. Yes, Memorial.
> S: Ah. Memorial Hospital.
> P: Yeah. And, ah, he put me in a hospital, Higgins, who's an arthritis specialist. My doctor sent me to him because I was very, very tired for one thing. I'd had a hard summer and I'd had a few more hard knocks and my neck had almost frozen in position because it hurt me so (rubbing hands, then hands to neck).
> S: Wow!

There's nothing wrong with using language that fits your personality. Not everybody would use the word "wow," but it fits Bill's style and clearly imparts to the patient that he understands how much her neck *hurts*.

> P: So he put me in a hospital and I had . . . it was good because I needed it. (Pauses.) I didn't want to admit that. And I had physical therapy twice a day.

Here is another casual aside—"I didn't want to admit that." Mrs. Walters says here, as she did earlier in her assertion that people could just learn to "ignore" her mistakes, that she doesn't like to let people in on how distressed she really is, how much pain she's feeling inside. This important disclosure about herself, however, is sandwiched between enough other medical facts that she is reporting to go by unnoticed.

S: I see.
P: Plus hot packs any time I wanted them. Which are really great. That's damp heat you see, wet heat.
S: Right. I'll bet that helped.
P: That helped. I still use that. And . . . (rubbing neck).
S: You do that every morning?
P: Yeah. At night and sometimes in the middle of the day if I have time . . . when I take the time. If I'm going somewhere, and it hurts very much today.
S: It does?
P: Yeah. Well I've been rushing around a lot this morning and driving the car, which means you turn your neck a lot.

Why has she been rushing around a lot this morning and driving the car? If one pauses to think about it, it's because she has been in a flurry of activity getting ready to come to be interviewed by Bill. This interview is important to her. Putting this together with what she has just said above about not wanting to admit to people when she is in pain, a picture begins to emerge on the process level. She is saying to Bill, "I don't like to admit to strong feelings, whether they be feelings of pain, fears about turning people off, or expressions of how important people are to me. But I did rush around a lot this morning to get here and this interview with you *does* matter to me, even if I try not to show it."

S: Right.
P: And ah . . . (sighing and shrugging shoulders).
S: Does it radiate down at all? (Student rubs his neck.) Or is it just in one spot?
P: It radiates up.
S: Way up in your head?
P: It goes up to my head so I think I must have a tumor up there. (Holds head.)
S: Oh no.
P: Sometimes I have an earache.
S: Earache? Do you have headaches or anything like that?
P: No. The earache is where it's hitting a nerve that's getting me back here, which seems to make my ear ache. No, it doesn't go down here at all (pointing to shoulder). It's here. It's right here.
S: Just in that one little spot.
P: Yeah, Well, what happens is, you see, it's got to be (rubbing other side of neck) from the backbone . . . it's pinching a nerve somewhere.
S: Hm. Hm. You can really feel that, then, huh?
P: Yeah. That's why it hurts some.
S: Does it go away during the day? When you put these hot packs on?
P: During the day? No, it doesn't go away with hot packs; it just feels better.
P: It feels better?

Repeating the Patient's Words

The psychologist, Carl Rogers, first introduced the technique of repeating the last few words of what a patient says to encourage the patient to open up. Some interviewers can get carried away with it, building whole "schools" of interviewing based on nothing but repeating what the patient says. This, of course, is ridiculous. But repeating the patient's words *can* be a very effective way of indicating interest and involvement in what the patient is saying. Equally effective are simple nods of the head, quietly saying "Hm-Hm," or just an attentive, concerned silence. Students who do this excessively will quickly turn a patient off, but Bill uses this technique in a most appropriate manner. One gets the definite feeling in this interview that as the rapport between Bill and Mrs. Walters is developing, Bill is more comfortable being silent and receptive and simply following what she is trying to communicate. Students initially tend to be uncomfortable with remaining silent. Silent attentiveness, however, is one of the most potent tools that an interviewer can use.

P: Yea. And then when you stop using the hot packet you can move your head a little better (moving neck side to side). Now if I tell you that last summer I wasn't moving my head you can see what the therapy did.

S: Couldn't move at all? You're doing really well.

P: Yeah.

S: Good. Excellent. But you say your hands are getting a little . . . (moving his fingers).

P: Well yeah. My hands . . .

S: It really doesn't seem like it has affected you because you just sort of go on with it.

P: Yeah. I keep going. Well, . . . doc . . . ah . . . you will find that some people do, you know, and some people don't. I have too many interests to stop (rubbing hands). (*Author's note:* Note that the patient begins to refer to the student as doctor.)

S: Yeah. You sound like it. That's great.

P: So I have to, you know . . . I either can sit down and say I'm an invalid or I can keep going. (*Author's note:* Such expressions usually indicate that a patient is in stage three of illness, the stage of reorganization.)

S: There's no way.

P: No.

S: You play an instrument, that's great that you keep that up.

P: Yes. I like that very much and I'm trying to get a lot of papers of my own in order at home and I don't know that I want to stay in Colorado the rest of my life . . . it's cold (stiffening neck).

S: Yeah, does that hurt? On a day like today?

P: Well, I think it does, but I am not positive that that really has anything to do with it. I got a lot of literature and I meant to look at it and see . . . I don't know. It hurt terribly last summer when it was so hot.

S: In the warm weather, huh?

P: Yeah . . . so . . .

S: Do you live alone?

P: Yeah.

S: You do?

P: Well, I have a cat.

S: You have a cat.

P: I had two cats and one died last summer and that sent me into a state of shock. Um . . .

S: What happened?
P: My cat? Well, he had that cat blood disease, it's like ... oh ... anyway, there's no cure for it. So he died and I knew he was going to but I wasn't prepared for it and it really shocked me.
S: I bet.
P: I just said, God, that's enough. You've done enough to me now, don't you take my cat and I really ...

The patient's process communications here are very poignant. Bill has become increasingly sensitive to her and in touch with her feelings in this part of the interview. When he asks her if she lives alone, she tells him the story of her cats. Clearly these cats were very important to her. On a process level, she is also saying something about loss in general, about her pain and despair over all the things that she feels have been taken from her—her health, her husband, her independence. "I just said, God, that's enough. You've done enough to me now ... " Another process communication in this material is very subtle, as process communications can sometimes be, but worth noting: the death of her cat, which pained her so, occurred "last summer." Now, go back in the dialogue eight lines and look at what she is saying. They had been talking on a purely "medical" level about whether cold aggravates her arthritis. She then says "I don't know. It hurt terribly last summer when it was hot." No one would expect an interviewer to pick up routinely on this kind of subtlety; but is it possible that the patient is communicating something very important? That her arthritis flared up, not because of the temperature, but because of an important emotional loss?

Bill very sensitively here sticks to the process level of Mrs. Walter's communications—the pain of facing life alone. As the interview resumes, watch how he responds.

S: Is it hard for you to live alone? Can I ask that? Or do you enjoy it?
P: Ah ... I have always enjoyed a great deal of being alone. I don't mind being alone a great deal, but I don't like late afternoon to come ... there's no one to have a drink with. Or anything like that.
S: Sure. (*Author's note:* Another simple, empathic remark that communicates to the patient that Bill understands and cares.)
P: So I don't even feel like having my usual cocktail. I watch TV or maybe I work until it's dark.
S: Do you belong to any social societies where you go out and play music with other people or anything like that?
P: No ... (rubbing and folding hands, rubbing ankle, folding hands). I don't know many people here because it's not my place. I've met a few people in volunteers but that's just while you're here, and I go to a church, but again, I don't have my car anymore ... I left it back East with my son. I haven't gotten it back ... he says it's not in good shape so I just use my daughter's once in awhile. And not having a car is rough. So I really couldn't afford it now. My whole lifestyle has changed, that's what bugs me.
S: I see. Do you have a daughter?
P: She's here. That's why I'm here.
S: How old is she?
P: Judy? She's in her early 30s.
S: 30s?

P: Yes. I have a son and another daughter. I have five grandchildren. My oldest grandson is 21.
S: I see. Well, they visit you, don't they?
P: They're in Long Island.
S: Ah huh.
P: And my daughter, oldest daughter, is in Palo Alto.
S: I see. Well you have a good sized family.
P: Oh yeah. Yeah.
S: Makes it good.
P: And I visit around, but as I say, my lifestyle has changed and I think that's the hardest of all.
S: How exactly has it?

Here is a very good example of how patients will repeat themselves until they are heard. In Mrs. Walter's discussion above, she'd talked about the difficulty of not having a car. She couldn't afford it and goes on to say she is living in Colorado because her daughter's here. In other words, this rather independent lady has been forced to become quite dependent. "My whole lifestyle has changed and that's what bugs me." The first time she says this, Bill does not pick up on the importance of this issue for her. Instead, he goes after more identifying data—"Do you have a daughter?"—which is fine, because patients will invariably give you another chance to understand them, especially when you have begun to establish a good rapport. So, 14 lines later, she repeats herself. And this time, Bill picks up on it:

S: *How exactly has it (changed)? (p. 130)*

Facilitation

Facilitation is purposeful encouragement to continue talking. Purposeful is the key word, implying direction and permission to talk at greater length. Facilitation is used to solicit additional information, i.e., "So what do you do? You said files."

Facilitation is also used to explore and assess a particular area, usually as one is prompted by a process clue. An example of this occurs on page 128.

P: *... and I'm trying to get a lot of papers in order of my own at home and I don't know that I want to stay in Colorado the rest of my life ...*

This leads Bill, almost intuitively, to ask:

S: *Do you live alone?*
P: *Yeah.*
S: *You do?*
P: *Well I have a cat.*
S: *You have a cat.*

P: *I had two cats and one died last summer and that sent me into a state of shock.*
S: *What happened? (p. 128–129)*

Analysis of the Midphase of the Interview

In this segment of the interview Bill has begun to settle into the interview with Mrs. Walters. He tracks with her statements more consistently. Going back over the dialogue in this part of the interview, listen to the smooth flow of their interchanges.

P: *I'm divorced.*
S: *You're divorced. (p. 125)*

P: *Type all the time.*
S: *And you type? (p. 125)*

P: *It radiates up.*
S: *Way up in your head. (p. 127)*

P: *. . . No it doesn't go away with hot packs; it just feels better.*
S: *It feels better? (p. 127)*

Several times in this part of the interview, Mrs. Walters has reintroduced the fact that the arthritis "hurts," and now Bill has started to listen, without running back to the identifying data.

P: *. . . and my neck had almost frozen in position because it hurt me so.*
S: *Wow. (p. 126)*

P: *. . . and it hurts very much today.*
S: *It does? (p. 127)*

P: *. . . it's pinching a nerve somewhere.*
S: *Hm. Hm. You can really feel that, then, huh?*
P: *Yeah. That's why it hurts some. (p. 127)*

P: *. . . it's cold (stiffening neck).*
S: *Yeah. Does that hurt? On a day like today? (p. 128)*

A theme is developed in this part of the interview that we suspect serves occasionally to buffer some of the emotional intensity they both feel but that Bill also uses nicely to share his understanding and to communicate his respect for an area of enjoyment and accomplishment in Mrs. Walter's life. The theme is music. Notice how it develops in this part of the interview and how it is used.

P: *. . . Most of my school training was music. Classical music . . .*
S: *Are you married?*
P: *I'm divorced. (Hand socks palm.)*
S: *You're divorced? So you were married while you were developing this but . . .*
P: *I've only been divorced a couple of years.*
S: *I see. Do you play an instrument?*
P: *I play the piano.*
S: *You do (with pleasure and surprise)! (p. 125)*

Here, Bill was initially shifting to safer ground. But clearly it led into another important area for Mrs. Walters—music—an area in which her self-esteem hasn't suffered, as it has in so many other ways.

P: ... *Lately those two fingers aren't doing their job ... they've lost their strength.*
S: *Does that cause any problems with your teaching at all (piano)? (p. 125–126)*

P: *I either can sit down and say I'm an invalid or I can keep going ...*
S: *You play an instrument, that's great you keep that up. (p. 128)*

P: *So I don't even feel like having my usual cocktail. I watch TV or maybe I work until it's dark.*
S: *Do you belong to any social societies where you go out and play music with other people? (p. 129)*

Bill's questions in this segment of the interview become less awkward, rambling, and more open.

P: *I had two cats and one died last summer and that sent me into a state of shock.*
S: *What happened? (p. 128–129)*

P: *... as I say my lifestyle has changed and I think that's hardest of all.*
S: *How exactly has it? (p.130)*

As Bill begins to explore beyond the arthritis and opens up—"What happened?"—the body language during the interview changes. Mrs. Walters folds her hands in her lap; the fidgeting, rubbing, and holding of her neck essentially stop.

Rapport has begun to develop. Bill has heard one major message even though it took a few tries, i.e., "it hurts." It hurts on many levels: there is physical pain, loneliness, and dependency. Bill has begun to pick up on these important messages. Rapport has also begun through Bill's recognition that Mrs. Walters has an area of strength and accomplishment—her music.

Let us return now to the interview (Mrs. Walters had been talking about the change in her lifestyle).

P: Well, I've always had money. (Leaves resting pose and resumes working hands.) I've always been able to do the things which were important to me. Now I don't. Period. I don't.
S: That does make for big changes.
P: And ah ... there wasn't ... to my way of thinking there wasn't any sound reason for that to happen so ... it shook me.
S: Hm. Hm. I see.
P: And I had a slight heart attack (rubbing neck) the first year I was here. I was in City Hospital. In fact, I was *put in* City Hospital. And the doctor that took care of me is my doctor now. He was a young intern then. Dr. Stevens. He's over at (the hospital across the street).
S: Hm. Hm.
P: And that's how I happened to come here. Both to work and to go see him—to go to the clinic.
S: Right.
P: And ... ah ... he sent me to a psychiatrist because he said my general tone was so ... alright, I'm alive and I'll keep going, but I'm not really interested.
S: Did you see that change at all?
P: He felt ... he didn't know me very well but he felt it very strongly. (Hands are quiet in lap.)

S: I see . . . ah huh.
P: And he said in his opinion I still had a great deal to give and to live for, and he wanted me to talk to someone.
S: Hm. Hm.
P: Well, oh, I didn't fight it either way.
S: Did you believe that at the time?
P: Oh yes, I knew he was right about that. But I didn't think I had let it show cause I can always put on a show. Anyone who's socially oriented can.
S: Sure.
P: And I didn't think that he was old enough and wise enough to notice it but he did and . . .

Here we see an excellent example of how patients talk in process about the here and now through displacement and also by talking about the present through the past. Mrs. Walters tells Bill the story about "a young intern." Though she put up a front, he was sensitive and perceptive enough to appreciate how she was feeling though she tried to "put on a show." And he was able to do this even though she worried at first that he wouldn't be "old enough or wise enough" to help her. She is talking here about Dr. Stevens, to be sure. But through this displacement, she is also talking about Bill. She is saying, in process, "Right now I'm getting the feeling that *you* are sensitive enough to understand me and help me even though you're young and inexperienced."

S: Do you think it helped?
P: Oh yes. A great deal. We didn't come to terms for a matter of months . . . the psychiatrist and myself . . . and after that it was just clear sailing and he did point out some of the things which had happened. Among other things he pointed out last summer about the cat, that it wasn't the cat I was mourning although I missed him, but I was mourning for all I had lost in the last six years. (*Author's note:* Notice how she now tells Bill directly what she has already communicated to him in process.)
S: Right. This was your divorce? And the other things that happened?
P: Hm. Hm. My home and so on and so forth. These things all . . .
S: That's very hard. (Bill is responding very empathically here.)
P: Yeah. (Sighs) They aggravate a condition which is there and undoubtedly they are what started to really aggravate my neck so much.
S: Bet that's possibly true.
P: Yeah. I'm sure this was all true. Trauma is very bad for anybody with arthritis. (Chuckles uncomfortably.) And ah . . .
S: Sure. Have you ever thought about teaching? (In the process, Bill gets a little uncomfortable here and shifts away to a "safer" subject.)
P: Yeah (rubbing neck). I did when I was younger but I was so busy doing so many other things and I tried to teach my kids . . . that was a failure . . . (bends over, massaging neck) so . . . they didn't want to learn in other words. No . . . I really don't . . .
S: Kids are hard to teach.
P: I'm not good at teaching, I guess, anyway.
S: How do you know that for sure though?
P: Well. I didn't even teach the girls much about keeping house in general and yet

I notice they do things the way I did, so I guess they copied.

S: Right.

P: Which maybe was teaching without my really knowing it but I think I'm a little impatient and you see when I started to take piano lessons I was only about 8, and I wanted to very, very badly, so no one ever had to say, "Practice."

S: Hm. Hm.

P: I was eager for it. Besides that was a long, long time ago. People were more appreciative of what they had. Indeed, I got up at 6:00 a.m. every morning to practice.

S: Really.

P: So I could get an hour and a half in before breakfast.

S: Did you have any recitals of any sort?

P: Oh yea. Sure. And then I went to a school up near Boston where we had a great deal of music and that . . . you know I knew I wasn't going to teach it or knew I wasn't ever going to be great but I was good and that's all I wanted. I didn't want any more than that. I've never been terribly ambitious.

S: What are you going to do now?

P: Well, just keep going. What else is there to do?

S: That's true.

P: I have my . . .

S: What do you mean by "keep going?" Do you have any real solid plans? Or ah . . .

Here is an example of how potent a tool the interviewer has when he is able to pick up on process communications. The patient sandwiched her communication in a commonplace cliché—"Well, just keep going"—and then quickly started to go on to another subject: "I have my . . . " Bill picked right up on this and brought her back, giving the concern the importance it really deserved: "What do you mean by 'keep going?'"

Observe how this facilitates her expression of important concerns as the interview continues.

P: You know, that worries me. Lately I haven't had any real solid plans. I've sort of stopped planning and let things happen.

S: Day to day sort of?

P: One day at a time, yes. (Chuckles.)

Up until now, Mrs. Walters had been talking about the past. Now, with Bill's help, she has begun to talk about her worries *right now*.

S: You still practice?

(Here Bill gets a little uncomfortable again and shifts back to music.)

P: Yes. I'm very apt to spend an hour just doing Czerny, because you don't think much while you're doing it. You just do it.

S: Excuse me?

P: Czerny. It's an exercise. (Moves hands as though playing piano.) He was a German. There were several of those, matter of fact. Czerny, he just wrote exercises which are beautiful and some of them are very very hard.

S: I see.

P: If you do Czerny, your mind is completely on what you are doing, and it doesn't go lilting off about what are you going to do later or anything . . . your mind's on that.

(A knock on the door signals student to begin closing the interview.)

S: Ah huh.

P: So it's a very good exercise.
S: This is for all parts? Is it just for your hands? For dexterity?
P: Yeah, dexterity. (Patient reaches for purse and puts it over her shoulder.) Czerny was a pianist, oh, probably 150 years ago.
S: I see.
P: And all he wrote was exercises, but some of them, for the hands, I mean exercises on the piano.
S: I see.
P: And people do violin and all the rest of it but Czerny ... some of Czerny's things are like sonatas even, they're beautiful, they're wonderful. I love Czerny (making a sweeping gesture with hand on chest).

The patient is talking about Czerny. But in displacement, on the process level, she is probably saying something about how meaningful it has been for this proud but lonely woman to make contact and establish a rapport in the present with Bill.

S: That is interesting. I don't know a lot about music and that was interesting.
P: Oh ... well.
S: Thank you very much. (Patient and student stand and shake hands.)
S: How did you spell your last name?
P: W-A-L-T-E-R-S, Martha Walters. And because I'm mad, I just say Martha M. Walters (gesturing in a sweeping theatrical manner) and I will not sign Ms. or Mrs.
S: Okay (chuckling). Thank you for letting me talk to you. I enjoyed it.
P: Yes, I enjoyed it too.

Empathy

Empathy, to which we have referred many times in this book, is participation in the thoughts and feelings of another. In this definition, *participation* is the key word, implying that the thoughts and feelings of the patient are registered and sustained so that understanding develops. Empathy does not imply complete identification with the patient, however. This distinction is made, because empathy is too often understood in distorted fashion to mean identification—you "should become" the other person, you "should be able to have" the same feelings in the same way with the same intensity, as the other person. This distortion of purpose often leads students to feel frightened, artificial, and inept in dealing with patients and their feelings. Empathy is hearing and appreciating the merit of what is being said, letting the patient know the student knows what his distress feels like.

Rapport

Rapport is a state of mutual trust and respect that allows for direct and open communication. Rapport is essential for effective interviewing and forms the basis of the growing doctor-patient relationship.

The terms empathy and rapport are frequently used interchangeably. We make a distinction in an attempt to give students some guidelines for understanding rapport in a clearer fashion—what constitutes rapport and what may be missing in the interview if rapport is not established.

Rapport is created when trust and respect are established—when the patient decides that what he or she says is being heard and tolerated (trust) and when the patient feels that the student is appreciating and understanding the many different facets of the patient's feelings and concerns (respect).

The experience of empathy is the most striking and obvious force in the establishment of rapport. Steady, comfortable eye contact and attentive, appropriate posture are others. As was mentioned in Chapter 5, style of dress and appearance are also significant in establishing rapport.

Rapport is necessary for the patient to feel comfortable enough to reveal the truly sensitive side of his concerns. Inexperienced students sometimes fail to appreciate that fact, plunging headlong into the "heart" of the matter, then wondering why the patient seemed so guarded and unavailable. Some students needlessly fear the sensitive areas, not appreciating that an atmosphere can properly exist for expressing them. As this interview shows, a patient almost spontaneously reveals the sensitive and poignant parts of his or her life when given the chance. This is, after all, the patient's expectation of what the doctor-patient relationship should encompass.

This final segment of the interview runs smoothly—it "clicks." Mrs. Walters talks spontaneously and in a more relaxed manner. There is a decrease in her physical activity. Bill Green is also less active. His comments are short, his questions less rambling and awkward and more to the point.

In taking a thorough medical history, Bill Green would have learned that Mrs. Walters had had a heart attack. He might have learned about her psychiatric care, if he had specifically asked about it. Patients are frequently reluctant to reveal a history of psychiatric treatment because they feel embarassed and in some cases fear being misunderstood by the "medical" doctor. Indeed a history of psychiatric care can lead to premature diagnostic biases that often are not warranted, such as "this patient basically has emotional problems," "this patient is depressed and needs tranquilizers," or "someone else (i.e., the psychiatrist) is basically responsible for this patient's care." None of these statements is true of Mrs. Walters. Bill has obtained a good picture of the nature and outcome of Mrs. Walter's psychiatric treatment, which should be part of any physician's understanding of this patient.

In the atmosphere of rapport that has been established, Mrs. Walters levels about herself. A separate story about her emerges as the interactions, thoughts, and feelings of this interview are put together. If Mrs. Walters were relating the story directly, it would go something like this:

> When I first came to Denver, I had a young doctor who took care of me. He took such good care of me that I decided to stay here in Denver. I even live close to his office. This doctor could tell I needed to be hospitalized for a slight heart attack, and he put me there. He could tell I needed to talk to someone, and he got me there too. He could tell I'm worthwhile and told me so. That's pretty good, because I'm used to putting on a show for people. You, Bill Green, remind me of my doctor. I slipped and started to call you "doctor" a while ago. You can tell I find the arthritis painful. And you must think I have musical talent—you keep suggesting I teach piano.

chapter 7

AFTER THE INTERVIEW

THE REHASH

In our interviewing course at the University of Colorado, each group of students and their preceptor get together after their patient interviews for a rehash. The group consists of four students and one preceptor. Often they meet for an hour or more, and over a 6 to 8-month span of weekly meetings, they usually become close to each other. We feel that every interviewing experience should be structured to permit time afterwards for discussion. It is ideal when these discussion groups can be small and their work extend over a significant span of time. This encourages an atmosphere of openness and trust to develop that we believe is important for an effective interviewing learning experience.

There are a number of specific functions that the rehash performs.

Ventilation and Sharing

An afternoon of interviewing patients can be an intense experience. Afterwards, students have an abundance of questions about the patient, about their performance, about technical matters of interviewing style. In addition, they often have strong feelings in response to interview subjects and events. They have been anxious in anticipation. The interview itself may have been difficult and intense. The rehash provides an opportunity to ventilate and share. Just as a runner needs to walk a few hundred yards to cool down after a race, students need an opportunity to wind down after an interview.

Elucidating the Process of the Interview

Usually, after students have been able to wind down, it is possible for the group to review the interviews and make some sense out of the process. In this area, a skilled preceptor can be very helpful. Integration of the process can take place on a number of levels. Sometimes the group may focus on observational data.

> A very loquacious middle-aged woman with blue tinted bouffant gray hair spent the first 3 minutes of the interaction talking to her friend on the telephone. She would not hang up, yet every time the student tried to indicate that they could leave and return later, she would beckon the group vigorously toward her with her hand.

From this observation, the discussion of process focused on three possible meanings: the patient's need for control, her need for constant contact with people, and the angry way in which she chose to express this through her process.

In other situations, the process of the interview may be discussed in regard to the emotions it evoked.

> A medical student was interviewing a 65-year-old hospitalized woman in the presence of her three classmates and preceptor. The patient had suffered from a myocardial infarction. The student was taking a medical history and the patient had been answering questions in a matter-of-fact way. She had seemed preoccupied and unanimated. The student then learned that the patient was a widow. Her husband had died a year and a half ago of a cerebral hemorrhage. Upon disclosing this, the patient started to sob. The interview seemed to grind to a standstill. While the patient cried silently, the student looked helplessly at her hands, then up at the ceiling, then at her fellow students and preceptor. After a moment or two, though it felt like an eternity to the student, the preceptor approached the bed and put her hand on the patient's arm. She said, "You must still miss your husband very much. It's still hard to talk about his death." The patient nodded. The preceptor then asked, "Do you have children?" The patient began to talk with more animation about her family, where they lived, and what they were doing. By the end of the interview, she had become animated and was smiling frequently as she discussed the activities that she would resume upon discharge.

The process in this interview centered on emotion—the lack of it at the outset, then the intense outpouring of grief, and finally the emotions this aroused in the students. The student interviewer initially felt worried, troubled in the rehash. She said, "I made her cry. I caused her pain." All four students then discussed the emotions that had surfaced during the interview. The preceptor pointed out to them that, at the outset, one of them had been staring out the window and another had been fiddling aimlessly with his stethoscope. The students acknowledged that they initially felt quite detached. The preceptor asked if they mightn't be reacting in some way to the patient's initial detachment and withdrawal. The students then recalled some of the thoughts that had gone through their minds as they seemingly daydreamed and couldn't pay attention. One of them remembered wondering what would happen if the patient started to cry. Later, when she did, his first reaction had been, "Let's get out of here!"

Thus, in this interview, the students were able to make sense of the interview process by examining their feelings. The initial detachment that they felt reflected the patient's wish to avoid her own underlying grief and pain. Yet, because the grief was there, there was a tension in the air, a sense of vague apprehension. This, they could see, was heralded by—of all things— one of their daydreams. One of the students had wondered, "what if she starts to cry?" Finally, from the same student's impulse to "get out of here," they decided that the patient might have similar feelings—wanting to get completely away from her own grief.

Finally, the students and preceptor spent some time acknowledging how helpful the patient's catharsis had turned out to be. For it was after she cried that her affect became more animated and her thoughts turned toward the future. One student asked, "Could the course of this little interview actually parallel what she has ahead of her in the next few months?" He went on. "I mean, at the beginning, she's tense and isn't focusing on anything. Maybe that's because she hasn't grieved as much as she needs to. Then she got some grief out. After that she felt freer to go on with the interview. Maybe the same thing will be true in her life if she can get those feelings out more." This was an excellent summary of the process.

In the rehashes, students become progressively more adept at identifying and making use of the seemingly trivial: a magazine article that lies open on the bed, reluctance to get off the phone, a mood in the room, a fantasy that one of the students has while he seemingly isn't even paying attention. In coming to appreciate the value of these elusive yet all important data, students begin to develop a deeper understanding of process and their excitement often grows. Part of the task over time is to help students recognize what they would ordinarily dismiss as being too vague, scientifically meaningless, "far-out," or peculiar. One group of students summed up their experiences in a successful interviewing course: "It's the use of feelings in the interview that's important and we're glad we learned that this year. If something is going on in the interview, there's a reason for it. Now we know that when we feel angry it may have something to do with the patient or what is going on between us. Earlier in the course, we were so wrapped up in ourselves and the content issues of the interview: were we asking the right questions?, did we remember all the points of the history? It wasn't until we got beyond this that we could begin to deal with the process."

The students were asked whether they felt it was possible to learn process at an early point in their training. They believed it was, if the concepts were actively elucidated and if some of their initial anxieties about "getting all the data" could be alleviated. Perhaps it would be more accurate to say that their definition of what constitutes valid data needed to be expanded to include process.

The Importance of Beginnings

In elucidating the process of an interview, it is worth making special note of the importance of beginnings. Often the most important data of all appear during the first few seconds of the interchange. Does the patient eagerly sit forward in bed and reach out with her hand or does she continue yakking on the telephone? Does the patient make exclusive eye contact with the interviewer, or does he tend to scan the room from person to person? Or does he fail to make eye contact at all? What is the significance of the casual aside, "I hope you'll pardon my appearance" or "It sure took you long enough to get here." As we discussed in Chapter 6, these "asides," when the student and patient feel they are "off camera," often disclose the most about the patient's underlying feelings and concerns. A similar function is served by the casual remarks that follow after an interview has officially ended.

In the beginning, until the student has trained himself to be especially vigilant to the details of those initial few seconds, the preceptor can be helpful.

A 45-year-old cocktail waitress had been admitted to a public ward for liver failure and alcoholism. She discussed her medical history in an aloof and hostile manner. At one point she remarked to the male student who was interviewing her, "You've probably seen a hundred like me, so why make me your guinea pig? Gals like me are a dime a dozen." In obtaining a social history, the student learned that the patient had been married and divorced four times. "All four of them were no good."

The student recognized that this woman was depressed and troubled, yet he had trouble understanding the patient's hostility toward him.

The preceptor asked, "Do you remember the first thing she said?" "Yes," the student said. "She said I'm here because of alcoholic liver disease."

"*Was* that the first thing she said?" the preceptor asked.

Then, another student recalled, "She did say something before that, something like—Oh boy, here comes another one."

From this small piece of data, the students were able to make many interesting speculations. This woman had been abandoned by four men, at least as she saw it. Could the remark "Here comes another" say something about her cynicism and apprehension about being abandoned now as well, by her doctors? Beyond this, could it even say something about a basic distrust toward everyone, which this patient brought to her view of life?

Speculation

An example such as the one above will often raise in many students' minds questions about the role of speculation in clinical thinking. Frequently during a lively session, students and preceptor alike will engage in a considerable amount of speculation. Often, from fairly limited data, they will have many ideas, hypotheses, and hunches about what is going on with the patient. Could the abdominal pain be the first sign of an ulcer, or might it be an early indication of gallbladder disease? Did the patient's reticence indicate some hostility? Or was she simply quiet, sad, and depressed? Or might her mind have been somewhere else entirely?

The role of speculation in medicine is important. Speculation is the basis of hypothesis generation and the capacity to generate multiple evolving hypotheses about a patient's illness over time is one of the hallmarks of clinical expertise. The emphasis placed in medicine on the concept of differential diagnosis is one clear example of this. The thoughtful physician is one who is able to think on several levels at once rather than setting his sights in a monocular manner toward one conclusion only. The experience of speculating, of allowing one's mind to wander, even to notions that at first seem a bit preposterous or extreme can be very valuable for students. An overly inclusive mind is preferable in medicine to a prematurely constrictive one. With experience comes the ability to prioritize one's hypotheses and speculations so that the clinician has a sense of their rank order, their relative likelihood.

By and large, the function of speculation in the rehash, therefore, should be expansive, encouraging the students to entertain broader notions and more expansive ideas about the data they observe. At the same time speculation has its hazards. First, some clinicians may get careless and base their speculations on what they think are data but which in fact are other speculations in their own right. Therefore, during the rehash, students should be aware of what is objective evidence (the data) and what is speculation. Confusion of these two can result in a great deal of muddied clinical thinking. Beyond this, there is a hazard if the clinician loses his own sense of critical skepticism about the speculations he generates. One obvious example of this in interviewing would be the student who has a strong reaction to a patient and jumps speculatively to the conclusion that this must automatically represent a countertransference to his patient's transference. It might also be that the student was having a strong reaction for other reasons, some entirely his own.

The reader may at times, in fact, have objections to speculations that we make in this book. Some speculations he may find himself agreeing with, others may seem a bit far fetched. This kind of skeptical stance is important in medicine and finds its highest expression in the clinician who can allow himself to entertain hunches but also regard himself with a very skeptical stance. Generally, we have found that students tend to inhibit speculation more than they over indulge themselves in it. Nevertheless, the maintenance of a sense of critical reserve—the willingness to entertain a hunch but ultimately expect a proof—these are the characteristics of the physician toward which we all must strive.

Discussion of Technical Issues

The rehash also serves as a forum for the discussion of technical issues and concerns that can range from the quite specific to the very broad. It is usually the context in which specific aspects of interviewing technique can most fruitfully be discussed. Advance lectures on the importance of eye contact, open-ended questions, and proper posture usually have limited meaning to students. On the other hand, it can be a powerful learning experience for a student to realize that he conducted his whole interview peering into a notepad, that he frequently interrupted his patient with leading questions, or that he did not permit periods of silence.

Videotape technology can make a contribution here. Such technology is probably not essential to the learning of interviewing skills. In fact, at times we feel it has been overrated at the expense of good bedside teaching. Nevertheless, a well timed videotape can be valuable. Students can see their mannerisms, posturing, and styles of inflection, often for the first time. The timing of videotapes seems to be important. Students have complained that when they make them too early in a course the effect can be demoralizing. The student does indeed see how anxious he appears. He becomes glaringly aware of nervous mannerisms that he displays under stress. Yet, if exposed to this prematurely, the student feels an understandable sense of helplessness, not knowing to what use he can put these observations. Generally videotapes are most useful for students later into their interviewing experience, when their confidence and sense of style have increased.

The rehash is also an appropriate environment in which to discuss more general questions of style and technique. For instance, the act of touching a patient has led to lengthy, animated discussions among our students about the pros and cons of physical contact in the doctor-patient relationship.

If the learning alliance in a group is proceeding well, one often notes a tendency for discussions to become increasingly free and broad-ranging. One week the group may focus at length on a particular patient. Other weeks the patients interviewed may not be discussed much at all. The students may wish instead to learn more about an area of pathophysiology or anatomy. Or they may want to know more about the preceptor and his areas of interest. Sometimes students may wish to share feelings and concerns of their own.

To an outsider, this may appear to be little more than a bull session; occasionally students worry about this themselves. Medical education is usually so structured and content bound that students may feel almost guilty about spending an hour or two talking about whatever is important to them in an atmosphere of mutual support and trust. On the one hand, they feel good about it and it seems to enhance their sense of self-awareness as professionals, yet they feel uneasy—how did they get into talking about such things anyway?

Actually, what goes on in such discussions is much more than a bull session. The students are actively experiencing a process akin to the doctor-patient relationship itself. When one follows these groups over time, an evolution can be discerned: phases of trust develop that parallel the evolution of a good clinical relationship. In the beginning, students are somewhat guarded, cautious about what they disclose, not sure exactly what is appropriate to bring up and how the course will proceed. As empathy and rapport develop, students feel increasingly comfortable sharing with each other and their preceptor, just as trust develops over time in the doctor-patient relationship. Finally, anyone who has witnessed the poignancy and power of feeling that students exhibit when these groups end will appreciate that something very meaningful has developed. This too has its implications for the doctor-patient relationship. It underscores in a very immediate way the importance that a physician can have for his patient over time. The phenomenon we are describing is called the parallel process.

The Parallel Process

One definition of the parallel process has already been described above: the student experiences, through his growing trust in his teacher and peers, a relationship that is supportive, empathic, and growth promoting. This gives the student a vivid, first-hand understanding of the ideal doctor-patient relationship itself, in which a similar process unfolds.

A second definition of parallel process has to do with the more focal phenomenon of a group's mood or interaction, which reflects the process of the interview that preceded it.

Beth was interviewing a painfully cachectic 52-year-old Hispanic male named Mr. Rodriguez. Mr. Rodriguez had been a patient on the general surgical ward for over 2 months. His sad story had begun with a rather simple operative procedure to correct a gastric ulcer. Then the problems had set in: infections, wound-dehiscence, hemorrhaging, electrolyte imbalance.

Two months, and several emergency surgeries later, Mr. Rodriguez remained on the ward, some 30 pounds thinner than he had begun, a glum symbol of medical failure and personal depression. Though Beth tried valiantly to strike up a relationship with Mr. Rodriguez, nothing she did seemed to help. He would heave great sighs and complain, "No, that wasn't it at all. That's not what I meant at all."

Afterwards, the students felt withdrawn and restless. One of them joked about "knocking off early today, or at least let's have the session out on the lawn." The preceptor attempted to engage their interest in every way he could think of. He drew diagrams on the board of the difference between Bilroth I and II procedures. He talked about the hyperalimentation Mr. Rodriguez was receiving. He discussed psychological dynamics. No matter what he did, the only responses he got back were bored looks and disgruntled yawns.

The group was engaged in a parallel process. Just as Mr. Rodriguez had made it clear to Beth that nothing she could do would be right, so the students in parallel process gave the same message to their preceptor. When the students realized this, one of them asked a rather sad question: Was it possible that the entire course of Mr. Rodriguez' illness too had been an expression of this same process? Could his failure to respond to one medical intervention after another reflect some deep-seated unconscious inability to improve?

The students, incidentally, were concerned enough about Mr. Rodriguez that they approached the surgery resident who was managing his care. Together, they decided to obtain a psychiatric consultation. The psychiatrist's evaluation disclosed the presence of a depression. A course of supportive psychotherapy and antidepressant medication was initiated. Within 1 month, Mr. Rodriguez gained weight, experienced considerable healing of his surgical wounds, and was able to return to his family. This rather dramatic chain of events underscores two points: First, the data that students obtain in their interviews can often be materially important to the clinical management of the patient. Second, the students recognized that their responsibility for their patient did not end with the completion of the day's interview but extended to obtaining follow-up. The importance of follow-up, to both students and patients, will be discussed more fully later in the chapter.

TRANSFERENCE AND COUNTERTRANSFERENCE

A group of students was watching a videotape of an interview conducted by a senior clinician with a young woman of 28. She had suffered for several years from multiple sclerosis. It was a moving tape, characterized by the perceptiveness of the clinician and the willingness of the patient herself to open up before the camera. Initially the patient described her first symptoms: numbness in her legs, sensitivity to heat when she took a bath, a pain in her right eye. At the beginning, she said, her reaction had been one of "puzzlement."

She had gone at first to an ophthalmalogist because of the eye pain. He referred her to a neurologist, a woman who had recently entered private practice. The patient said, somewhat emotionally, "She did a bunch of tests: coordination, reflexes, and the like. Then she said, 'Well, Gail, I think I want you to go into the hospital so I can do some more tests to confirm what I already suspect.' " The patient continued. "I asked her what that was and she said 'multiple sclerosis.' I said, what's that? The doctor said, 'A crippler of young adults.' "

Gail went on to talk about the relationship that developed between them. The doctor offered to follow her case, though Gail could not afford private fees, and suggested that she call every week to report on her progress. But Gail did not experience this as comforting. She resented the fact that her neurologist insisted on "keeping tabs on me, as though I were some kind of a dependent baby." Nevertheless, the relationship continued between them and the patient described it as being, on the whole, "very good—she really cared about me."

Then, 7 months into the treatment, she developed new symptoms and called her neurologist in a state of alarm. The patient recounted it this way: "I told her my symptoms. The doctor said 'That's sensory.' I thought to myself, 'What does that mean!! That's sensory'—as though that summed up everything. It didn't tell me anything. So, I told the doctor on the phone how annoyed I was getting. I said to her, 'I want some answers! All you give me are generalities. You're never specific.' Then, the doctor said 'Now, now, Gail, we've been through this before and we will be again.' That really annoyed me! Then her receptionist cut in and told me I had to get off the line."

At this point in the interview the patient's affect saddened. "The next day, when I called her back, she told me 'I think you'd better go to the Clinic at the University, Gail. I can't continue to treat you at reduced fees.' Gail went on, "That really hurt. I'd built up a sense of trust, only to be rejected. I think it was because I got angry at her—so she pushed me away."

The interviewer then asked, "Have you had any contact with her since?"

"No," Gail tersely replied.

The interview stirred up a lot of reaction. Several students commented on the pathos and valor of this young woman who had gone on to accept further treatment and had continued, with the help of some psychotherapy, to function very effectively as a wife and mother of two.

As for Gail's strong reaction to her doctor, the group seemed divided. Some of them readily took her side. They felt that the neurologist was dumping her on a public clinic when the going got rough. They responded to her account as another example of how insensitive doctors can be to their patients. Another group of students reacted differently. They were more timid initially, but eventually spoke up. They saw things quite differently. They were struck with Gail's whiny, demanding quality.

"What does she expect?" one student asked with some irritation. "Perfection?"

The student went on to point out the many things that Gail's doctor had done right. She had offered to spend time supporting Gail emotionally. Another student could not understand why Gail was annoyed with the doctor's offer to keep in close contact with her by phone. Furthermore, this same student pointed out, the doctor had invited Gail's husband in at the outset of the evaluation and encouraged them to share their feelings and questions with her. Thus, the second group tended to see Gail as irrationally demanding of perfection and, on top of that, "a bit of an ingrate."

The argument went on. After a while, the preceptor resumed showing the videotape. It was a later section of the interview. Gail was talking about her mother.

"I never felt that I could win her love and approval. I remember when I was 10, my mother called all of us kids together. She was drunk—often the case. She put each of my brothers on her lap, kissed them, and told them she loved them. Then she invited me to sit on her lap. I could smell the whiskey on her breath. I sat on her lap and she bent forward like she was going to kiss me, then she pushed me off onto the floor and screamed, 'I hate you!'" There were tears in Gail's eyes as she went on. "I knew what she was going to say next. She reminded me that I had been named after my sister."

The interviewer asked for clarification.

"Well," Gail went on, "there had been another girl born a couple of years before me. She had the same name as me. She died when she was 3 days old. My mother named me after her, but she always told me that I never measured up. I was never as pretty or as smart."

"It must be pretty hard sometimes to tell who *you* really are," the interviewer said, "if you're always trying to be someone else—your dead sister, the one who got your mother's love."

This vignette illustrates the concepts of *transference* and *countertransference*.

Transference technically refers to those reactions and behaviors toward significant people from the past that are (unconsciously) carried over and reenacted with a figure in the present. It is as though the object of the transference reaction and behaviors is not a person in his own right but rather the reincarnation of some unknown figure from the past. Anna Freud, addressing a class of medical students at Case Western Reserve University, summarized what happens in transference this way: "Evidently (the patient) has turned the doctor into someone else."

Gail's reaction to her neurologist was a transference, based on her feelings toward her mother. The fact that the neurologist was a woman no doubt helped hurry this reaction along, though it is entirely possible that Gail might have ended up perceiving a male doctor this way as well. Probably, Gail's intense anger toward her neurologist for "not giving me the answers" was a displacement of anger toward her mother for never giving her the love she needed. When the neurologist, doubtless exasperated, referred her to the University clinic, Gail felt as though once again she had been rejected, pushed from her mother's lap.

The reaction of the students, on the other hand, and probably Gail's neurologist as well, were instances of countertransference. Countertransference is a physician's emotional reaction (again largely unconscious) to the transference of the patient. But, as we can see, countertransference is also shaped considerably by the temperament and biases of the individual experiencing it. In this example, we can discern different responses to the same patient's transference. The neurologist, in all likelihood, responded initially as a protective loving mother, wanting to make up for the deprivations she sensed in her patient's past by nurturing her and protecting her— "Call me every week." When the patient got angry (a negative transference), the perplexed neurologist probably felt guilty, as though she had failed personally. At this point, she washed her hands of the case.

Among the students, the group who stuck up for Gail probably had a countertransference similar to the one that the neurologist initially displayed. On the other hand, another group of students responded to Gail as an angry, demanding infant who seemingly could not be satisfied, who should learn how to behave.

Generalized Transference

Transference occurs in all relationships. In the special relationship of psychotherapy, the vicissitudes of transference can become a major focus of treatment. In the majority of medical interviews, however, issues of transference and countertransference are rarely focused on specifically. Although transference is always there, it seldom emerges with a force that calls much attention to it. For instance, every doctor notices that patients respond differently to him as a symbol. Some patients react with deference, others with overidealization. Still others seem defiant, as though the physician, as an authority figure, must be challenged. These are what might be called generalized transferences. They are the unconscious, repetitive expectations from the past that the patient automatically endows every figure with in the present. Thus, to cite one extreme example, for the bar room brawler, every cop, every bartender who says it's time to close, every authority figure is "a _____ who ought to be socked in the nose."

Specific Transference

Beyond general transference, however, there is another phenomenon that develops more subtly as a relationship deepens over time. This is specific transference. We see this clearly in Gail's gradually emerging relationship with her neurologist. The relationship was initially cordial and founded in reality. Slowly, however, Gail began to confuse her neurologist with her mother. When her feelings about her mother erupted suddenly in the form of her response to the doctor, it took everyone by surprise.

If a clinician is unfamiliar with the existence of transference, as perhaps Gail's neurologist was, its manifestation can seem highly perplexing. Often when transference erupts, the clinician searches in vain for some "rational" explanation to explain this behavior. Of course, none is readily apparent, because the rational explanation is locked in the patient's past, unbeknownst to physician and patient alike.

Over time, students will repeatedly become the object of both general and specific transferences. At the outset, when their contacts with individual patients are usually brief, for the most part they will encounter general transferences. These are displayed by patients whom clinicians label as "angry," "dependent," or "seductive." Such patients have general transferences to everyone in the present, which compel them to react in stereotypic, monotonously repetitive ways to every new person they meet, including the doctor. These patients can be troublesome, but usually they are less befuddling to the clinican than those who develop a specific transference.

Yet, if students allow themselves to get close to their patients over time, specific transferences will also emerge. Recall the relationship between Paul and Mrs. Clark in Chapter 1. At one point, Paul felt he was too busy with school work to make it to one of their appointments. At the time, Paul had hardly thought it would matter. Yet, to Mrs. Clark, it turned out to matter greatly. She expressed considerable hurt and disappointment, the magnitude of which surprised Paul and made him feel a little confused and off balance. For that matter, one might consider whether Paul's not going to an appointment or two represented his countertransference. Mrs. Clark's transference was intense, though neither of them was fully aware of it. She was saying, on an almost unconscious level, "You're becoming very important to me. I need you a great deal. I depend on you." This probably frightened Paul, so he backed off and had a countertransference, expressing his dilemma through his actions rather than through words: "It scares me to be so important. I think I'll not show up. Maybe that will be a way of telling you to cool it a bit. Don't expect more from me than I'm able to deliver."

Transference in the Student

Not all emotional reactions to patients by students are countertransference. On the one hand, some are realistic. A student's admiration for a paraplegic who rehabilitates himself and enters a wheelchair marathon is not countertransference. It is respect. On the other hand, students can also develop transferences to their patients, and these are to be distinguished from countertransferences by their lack of relationship to the patient's way of relating.

Kevin was assigned to interview a patient with cerebral palsy. The patient had severely impaired gutteral speech and her physical motions were very spastic. When he walked into the room where she was sitting and saw her flailing her arms, he initially recoiled and stepped backward toward the door. He then drew forward and pulled up a chair. In a brusque voice he commanded the patient to "tell me your life history in 2 minutes." As the patient became confused and began to mumble more, Kevin became more irritated. "Well, where were you born, what do you do, where did you go to school, have you finished school, how long have you lived in Colorado, what do you do for a living?" He repeatedly interrupted the patient when she failed to get quickly to the point and at times argued with her about the accuracy of dates and facts that she gave.

This is transference on Kevin's part. He is not reacting to a patient's transference toward him, which would be countertransference. Rather the patient is stirring something up in him quite independently. In this case, it turned out to be a younger sister. In the rehash, Kevin became aware of his callousness, which was not at all typical of him. He somewhat bashfully wondered whether "it might have to do with the fact that I had a younger sister who was retarded." He went on to tell his group a bit about what it was like to have a sister, four years younger than he was, born with severe Down's Syndrome requiring early institutionalization in a home for the retarded. Kevin's unconscious feelings toward his sister became the focus of a transference toward his patient.

Effect of the Student's Background and Experience

Not all misperceptions of patients originate in a student's transference. Students usually begin their training with a limited number of experiences outside their own socioeconomic and cultural background. Yet patients from a very different background are typically the ones that students are expected to treat, especially in a teaching hospital. Students naturally do their best to understand their patients and just as naturally attempt to do so by drawing on experience from their own background and family and friends.
Here is an example:

A young female medical student, poised, and stylishly dressed in expensive clothes, was discussing discharge planning with a 56-year-old male patient who had been hospitalized for cirrhosis and malnutrition. The topic under discussion was what kind of activities, both work and social, the patient might undertake upon discharge. The patient shrugged his shoulders and sighed as he talked about having little structure to his life, having worked only marginally for the last few years. "I'm not sure I have much future anymore. I'm 56 years old now. I just don't seem to have any energy left." The student responded quickly "Oh, but Mr. Jones, 56 is not so old. My mother is 56 and she is very active." "Miss Baker," the patient wearily replied, "I think your mother has probably led a very different type of life than I have."

As a beginner, Miss Baker did not have a host of previous experiences to draw upon that would have helped her understand this patient, his behavior, and his symptoms. She had experiences of being intimately involved with people, as the physician is at some level with every patient, but not with anyone quite like this man. It is only through repeated contact with patients that the student develops a new, broader repertoire of experiences. Through repeated clinical exposures the "human family" gradually expands for the student. The evolution is a desirable process that hopefully every clinician goes through. Too often, however, we fail to appreciate many of the fine, human sensitivities that students first come with. We rather crudely dismiss such sensitivities, calling a student like Ms. Baker naive and expecting that she'll "wise up." Too often the sensitivities of medical students get simplistically categorized as being due to naivete and inexperience, too much idealism, excessive openness, almost as though we find it expectable, and desirable, that the student get callous. By understanding the perspective that beginning students bring to their interactions with patients, we can more easily help them move beyond their provincialism as time goes on and help them build upon important previous learning of value. By understanding and acknowledging where the student begins, we are less apt to make one feel "silly" for the first spontaneous interactions with patients, or worse yet, encourage the development of negative attitudes such as jadedness and cynicism.

Clinicians' Reactions to Transference and Countertransference

Clinicians who are unaware of transference and countertransference generally react to its manifestations with vexation, embarrassment, and a wish to sweep its signs and symptoms under the rug.

A 25-year-old male medical student in an outpatient clinic was interviewing an attractive but somewhat overly made-up young woman with systemic lupus erythematosis. Throughout the interview, he found himself distracted by her constant crossing and uncrossing of her legs, which revealed a considerable expanse of thigh. He even had some sexual thoughts, which made him feel guilty and ashamed.

Initially, in the discussion that followed, he kept these observations to himself. The preceptor then remarked on the patient's short skirt and seductive mannerisms. With this lead, the student felt more comfortable in admitting some of his sexual responses to her.

"That's very valuable data!" the preceptor said with enthusiasm.

Tom, a bit taken aback by the fact that his confession seemed to evoke such delight, asked for more explanation. The preceptor responded by pointing out how much Tom's reaction told them about the patient.

"After all," the preceptor said, "what must she have been trying to say? Her lupus has made her feel unattractive. She's got a big butterfly rash on her face, cold icy blue fingertips from Reynaud's Phenomenon. Her unconscious need to get you turned on was her way of trying to reassure herself— "I *am* still attractive."

Thus, the clinician who can become aware of transference and countertransference—and they are everywhere once you begin to look for them— has a very rich source of information about his patient. A good clue to the presence of transference and countertransference is the sudden eruption of intense emotions, in either the patient or clinician, that seem inappropriate in their timing or intensity to the context in which they arise. If a physician is not aware of the possibility that he is dealing with transference, his usual reaction is to back off. The patient's reaction seems irrational and therefore something to be stifled, ignored, and diverted. The clinician, if he is experiencing countertransference, may feel embarrassed and confused and try to push such thoughts out of his mind. If one can get beyond the initial wish to disown these reactions, they provide a rich vein of information about the patient and about the process that is unfolding during that patient's interaction with his doctor.

LEARNING ABOUT ONESELF

A group of students beginning a course in human behavior at the University of Colorado Medical Center expressed some misgivings about the small group format into which part of the course was organized. They wondered and worried whether weekly discussion groups consisting of eight students and two teachers, most of whom were psychiatrists, mightn't turn into "group therapy." Similar concerns about revealing oneself arise among students taking our interviewing course, though here the ratio is usually four students to one preceptor and frequently the preceptor is not a psychiatrist. Some students are more comfortable than others. But many students do, legitimately, raise the question of where to draw the line between experiential learning and "therapy." Some students are especially sensitive to the notion that they will be pressured into self-disclosure by their preceptor or peers.

One must acknowledge that these students have a point. Previously we discussed parallel process. This concept supposes a real, if imperfect, parallel between the doctor-patient relationship and the teacher-student relationship. Furthermore, we have made the point that experiential learning of this kind is as much emotional and personal as it is cognitive and content-bound. So, where does one draw the line?

Herbert Pardes, a psychiatric educator, describes his experience with a small group of medical students this way:

"The . . . thing that I came to realize was that one student no more represents all medical students than does one faculty member represent all faculty. There were people in that discussion group whose concerns ranged from how to get out of that small group as rapidly as possible, to how to ask a question about certain fears and personal problems they were having, to how to get a date for the weekend. They were all unique individuals with a multitude of different interests and concerns, not an "army of adolescents" seeking to prey on anything that looked like an adult or part of the establishment. Over the period of many months that the small group met, many of them, either within the group or privately with me, discussed personal worries, professional concerns, problems they faced with their families, reactions of all sorts generated by the lectures or reading material. The relief secured by this opportunity to discuss issues of personal concern which actively preoccupied them seemed to increase their comfort, and their ability to devote their full efforts to learning and developing their skills as beginning physicians. I believe this focus on the personal experiences of students, complemented by an atmosphere which encourages sensitivity to the individual needs and differences of both students and patients, can serve as an invaluable model for future physicians."

We agree. We concur especially with Dr. Pardes' notion that sharing feelings serves a definite educational purpose: increasing the student's comfort and mastery of material that he confronts as a beginning physician.

As much as many physicians may wish to deny it, medicine is an extremely stressful field. The very experiences that give the doctor's life such intense personal meaning—intimacy with patients, close contact with life in its most elemental forms, the intense joy and discovery that can occur when a patient invites us into his life—all of these can also cause us great distress. The horror stories about addiction, alcoholism, divorce, and suicide among doctors are well known. As one physician put it, "You could sum it all up by saying that we doctors have more of everything!"

The reasons why a doctor's joy can turn to vulnerability, or even disaster, are complex. One important factor, however, is the great stress physicians place on themselves to be totally omnipotent and self-reliant. Too often, the ideal physician is symbolized as a stalwart, self-denying "rock of Gibraltar," a lone soldier who never winces, never sleeps, never cries. One of the authors, when he considered a surgery residency during his medical school training, was told, "In this program, the divorce rate is 100%. You're on every other night. In the last 10 years no marriage has ever survived!" As hard as this is to believe, the person who told the author this said it with pride! Divorce, loneliness, and sleep deprivation seemed to symbolize for this resident a badge of courage, his medical "Purple Heart." Another resident in this same program told the author, "There's only one thing wrong with being on call every other night—you miss the chance to work up half the patients who come to the hospital."

In our view, this kind of mythology, which continues to pervade many areas of medicine, is not only destructive to the well being of the physician but also represents poor patient care. A study was conducted by the cardiologist, Friedman, in the late 1960s. In this study, Friedman had a group of interns read EKGs prior to being on call. He then had them read similar EKGs after having been up all night on call. Their overall performance was significantly worse in the latter circumstances, despite the fact that a monetary reward was given to those interns who performed the best. Yet, in most medical centers, inhumane call schedules have not changed. In our view, at least part of the explanation must be found in the irrational wish of many doctors to prove themselves invincible and omnipotent.

What does this have to do with opening up and learning about oneself in a small group setting? We believe, a great deal. Aside from the inherent pleasure that accompanies increased self-knowledge and new discovery, we believe that the physician who can share his feelings is a stronger physician. The tender physician is a more flexible and effective clinician than is the "rock of Gibraltar." A physician who is excessively afraid of his own feelings is bound to lack empathy for his patients.

In our experience, most small groups with experienced preceptors go well. Interestingly, where the disasters have occurred, the group leader was often the culprit. Students complained that he was too silent or analytic. The emotions that patient contacts stir up in all of us are intense. A mature preceptor is one who can freely express such feelings in himself as well as encouraging their expression in his students. Openness in the preceptor about his own feelings of vulnerability and his own experiences of stress as a student or physician can be very reassuring and meaningful to students. In addition, this openness helps preserve the educational and learning function of the group experience and prevents it from becoming group therapy. To this end, preceptors have an important responsibility to clearly remember the educational goals behind opening up and sharing. Being a student and learning about feelings is not the same as being a patient receiving medical treatment or psychotherapy.

COMMON LEARNING STYLES IN STUDENTS

Beyond the phenomenon of countertransference, which is a specific reaction to a certain patient on a particular occasion, some students tend to have characteristic interviewing styles. Occasionally these styles can pose learning problems for the student, and several are prevalent enough to warrant identification. Interviewing styles can be distinguished from countertransference by their stereotypy, repetitiveness, and inflexibility from patient to patient.

The Compulsive Perfectionist

This student has a great distrust of imprecision. He wants outlines, protocols, and specificity. He tends to be more comfortable with ideas than feelings and often manipulates these ideas into complex intellectualized constructs. He is not so much against feelings as he is anxious to be given an outline and checklist for identifying and categorizing them. Often such students take excellent content-oriented histories but have more difficulty assuming an open-ended empathic stance toward a patient.

> Mike, a highly organized and conscientious student, insisted on taking an outline with him to each patient interview. In addition, he took copious notes, often scribbling madly away at the bedside, asking the patient periodically to "slow down so I can get that point" and frequently failing to maintain eye contact. On one occasion, he conducted his interview with a diabetic patient, whose medical course was complicated, by flipping through pertinent sections of Harrison's *Textbook of Medicine*.

Although this sounds somewhat satirical in the telling, Mike was neither insensitive nor deliberately remote from his patient. He just found it very painful to immerse himself into the uncharted waters of the interview without some support—a notepad, outline, or textbook.

Usually, it is a mistake to expect such students to relax right away. A more helpful stance is to assist them to reduce their dependence on outlines and notetaking to more reasonable levels. Students and preceptors alike should remember that different students have different learning styles. The student who tends to be compulsive may have to be especially patient with himself because he develops an understanding of process more slowly. Also, students with this learning style often make excellent physicians. What they may lack in initial intuitiveness and sparkle, they make up for in thoroughness, conscientiousness, integrity, and a developed sense of responsibility.

The Emotionally Reactive Student

In some ways the opposite of the compulsive perfectionist, the emotional reactor tends to be intuitive, emotionally expressive, and demonstrative in his speech and gestures. He reacts to people, ideas, and situations intensely. He is often imaginative, and frequently comes from a premedical background in the humanities as opposed to the basic sciences. He often exudes warmth, anger, or sadness, depending on the situation. Whatever he feels, he always feels it strongly.

On the other hand, he may lack self-discipline. He tends to be somewhat befuddled by all the trivia he must memorize in medical school and often falls behind in his studies, indulging in last minute cram sessions. His approach to interviewing is enthusiastic yet sometimes lacks logic and a sense of appropriate objective distance.

> David was a junior medical student on his first surgery rotation when he worked up Ralph, a 26-year-old drifter and occasional ranch hand. Ralph had been admitted to the surgery unit electively for a partial gastrectomy due to chronic ulcers. He had been told by a doctor that he should admit himself for this

operation. He was also out of money, out of friends, and out of gas. When he was checked in at admissions, his belongings included a cowboy hat and fancy tooled leather cowboy boots which were polished to a lustrous sheen. What he failed to check in at admissions, which was later discovered under his mattress by one of the housekeepers, was a nearly empty flask of vodka.

David worked his patient up carefully and was intrigued by Ralph's many tales of adventure and hardship, which ranged from a "bad break" that landed him in the brig when he was in the military to a stint in jail for armed robbery. Nevertheless, David was taken by his outward charm and the many fascinating tales he told of life on the road.

However, the morning after admission, David returned to see his patient again. Ralph had overnight become belligerent, angry, and restless. His hands were tremulous. He demanded to be released from the hospital immediately, or "I'll bust somebody in the nose." David was so emotionally overtaken by this change of events that he failed to notice some important objective data. His patient's hands were tremulous. His pulse was also up and he had a slight fever. Most likely, his patient had gone into alcohol withdrawal.

After much arguing about the wisdom of staying in the hospital "just a little longer" the admission ended in a heated argument between David and Ralph at the elevator. Ralph had wrenched the i.v. line from his arm and hurriedly scrambled into his dungarees and boots. "I'm getting out of here and you ain't stopping me!" David beseeched, implored. Finally Ralph shoved him away, saying, "If you don't let me go now I'm gonna have to punch you in the nose, squirt." David backed off and Ralph stormed into the elevator and was never seen or heard from again.

When David turned around, he was chagrined to find the junior and senior surgery residents laughing at him. "Why did you care?" one of them asked mockingly.

No one would condone the way the residents treated David, but they had read his temperament accurately, however cruelly they chose to express it. David was so caught up in his emotional reaction to the situation, that he could not get enough distance to objectify his experiences. Had he done so, he might have noticed the alterations in his patient's vital signs, which would have alerted him to the possibility of an acute medical condition—here, alcohol withdrawal. Even if he had not picked this up, however, he still would have been in a better position to decide what to do. If his patient really needed to stay in the hospital, he could have called the hospital security police. Or, perhaps because the surgery was elective, it did make sense to allow Ralph to leave if he was so insistent.

The rigors of premedical education tend to eliminate a fair number of students who are primarily emotional reactors. The compulsive perfectionist is more likely to make it through the maze of premed requirements into medical school. Nevertheless, a sizable proportion of emotional reactors do join the ranks. Actually, the compulsive perfectionist and the emotional reactor may have more in common that meets the eye. Both, at different extremes, are having difficulty setting their "empath-o-stats." Unlike the more typical student, who vacillates between extremes, the compulsive perfectionist and the emotional over-reactor tend to settle consistently at one extreme of the dial or the other.

The Doer

The doer cannot stand still. Action specialties appeal to him: surgery, emergency medicine, orthopaedics. Enthusiastic, tireless, full of esprit de corps, the one response he finds intolerable is passivity. The student we cited earlier in the chapter who could not stand the pain of his arthritic patient's depression and dealt with this by rushing in with a barrage of small talk, jokes, and banter about bridge, may have been a doer. So is Gordon.

> Gordon was interviewing a 66-year-old black widowed woman who was in the hospital for heart failure and arthritis. Her tale was wrenching. Two of her sons were in jail. Her husband had disappeared 5 years previously.
> She had led a life of considerable suffering. She mentioned to Gordon that she was worried about losing her house. Because she had no insurance of her own and Medicare was insufficient to cover her bill, a social worker had told her that the county hospital might have to put a lien on her house—the one possession she owned outright after years of hard work as a domestic.
> Gordon was incensed. He said, "I've heard enough! That's ridiculous! I'm gonna call the hospital administrator myself, and if that doesn't work I'm gonna call Legal Aid and get you a lawyer!"
> The dumbfounded patient tried to suggest that perhaps such extreme actions were not yet necessary, but Gordon was not to be deterred. He terminated the interview abruptly and rushed off to attack the hospital bureaucracy with all the passion of Don Quixote charging full bore at the proverbial windmill.

Nobody would question the depth of Gordon's compassion and social zeal. Yet, here clearly was a student invoking the defense of action—doing seemed less painful than feeling.

Such students have a difficult time maintaining a receptive silence. They are often tempted to ask a lot of questions and "dig into the history" before the patient has finished his story. Often, in the group rehashes, these students are especially impatient with discussions that focus on interview process and the feelings of the patient. They are eager to get on with the "important stuff"—anatomy and pathophysiology or sociocultural issues.

Often, such students can master a more receptive stance once they see what a good, quietly empathic interview can do. When Gordon saw the benefit that patients experienced when they are able to open up, he commented, "I guess sometimes doing less can actually be more." Still, such students sometimes have a tendency toward a medically itchy trigger finger. They need to be aware of the tendency they have to *do for* a patient, sometimes in lieu of *being with* the patient.

Mr. Nice-Guy

This student is a special type of doer. He tends to be very active with patients and prefers to downplay emotions rather than encourage them. He often jokes with his patients and can often be seen clapping his patients on the shoulder, talking about the weekend football scores. He means well. But he fears that allowing patients to cry or focusing on their pain will make them feel worse.

Often seeing the benefits of allowing such feelings to come out during an interview is sufficient to convince this student that sometimes, in medicine, being therapeutic involves permitting the patient to experience and verbalize some pain.

The Skeptic

This student sometimes begins by thinking that interviewing courses, ICM, and human behavior courses are "basically fun but bullshit—this stuff is interesting, but what does all this really have to do with my being a doctor." He may or may not express this directly to his preceptors, but he is usually vocal about his opinions with his peers. He may also make his feelings known through a tendency towards silence, an unmistakable expression of skepticism, and, sometimes, a failure to show up.

Sometimes, the underlying problem of such a student is anxiety, although this is not always so. Often these students are not the most anxious but the brightest and most interesting. They must be won over with proof, at which point they have been known to become avid converts. Pardes cites his experience with one such student:

> For my initial session I met with some ten medical students ... After about fifteen to twenty minutes ... one student raised his hand and said in a rather cocky and defiant way, "Why the hell do you have to go to medical school to be a psychiatrist?" I was thrown not so much by the substance of the question as the tone. I felt an initial urge to fight back ... I mumbled and bumbled through various answers, all the while feeling that I was facing a tough questioner ... It took time for me to recognize what lay behind the question, and to realize that the dare of the question also signified a process of active questioning present within the interrogator. Later in the course, when he asked me with puzzlement, "How can you be an analyst?" I was a bit less thrown ... As the reader may have suspected, this student became a psychiatrist, and I last saw him at a meeting of psychoanalysts.

Obviously, the goal of an interviewing course is not to turn skeptics into psychiatrists but to help enhance their appreciation of process in themselves and their patients. Often those who are the most skeptical turn out to be the most enthusiastic, if we can teach with sufficient skill to convince them of our subject's value.

In many ways, the healthy skeptic is one who says, "Wait a minute, how do you know this is what the patient is thinking? Aren't you making too much out of this little piece of information?" What such a student is really saying through his questions is that this new way of looking at people and their behavior is foreign to his previous way of thinking about and understanding people. Such students are actively engaged in new learning. They are attempting to reconcile their old ways of understanding with new experiences, the essence of learning.

On the other hand, the skeptic who votes with his feet poses a more serious and troubling problem. The student who fails to show up repeatedly, who is silent and hostile in rehash after rehash may be struggling with serious anxieties that need to be confronted quickly and openly.

The Psychiatrist

Just as some students seem to know from the day they come to medical school that they're going to be neurosurgeons, some others "know" they want to be psychiatrists. The fact that students rarely stick to their early specialty choices is less important here than the fact that many of these students close themselves off defensively from certain types of learning experiences. The compulsive perfectionist, the doer, the skeptic—these students all tend to avoid affect in their patients. The "psychiatrist," by contrast, is comfortable with feelings but often resists obtaining a thorough medical history.

Karen was a 1st year student when she conducted a videotape interview with a 65-year-old woman. Karen's father was a prominent psychiatrist in town, and she also planned to be a psychiatrist. Still, the purpose of this videotape was to obtain a medical history and Karen expressed frustration. She said "Mrs. Henderson didn't really have much of a medical history, so I was able to do that part of the interview quickly and spend the rest of the time dealing with her depression."

When the videotape was played back, the following process emerged. Karen had begun by asking the patient what her medical problem was. The patient began to speak of a hospitalization earlier in the year for a hiatal hernia. In rapid succession Karen asked a series of questions about the hospital: how long was the patient there, how did she feel about it, how she was treated? Karen would respond empathically to an emotional expression from the patient, then flip through the pages of her tablet referring to an outline of points to be covered in the history of present illness.

She next asked about medication. The patient replied "Medication makes it worse. I take medication for my neck. I have arthritis."

"Is it hard for you having arthritis?" Karen asked. "You must not be able to move around as much as you'd like."

The patient commented that actually it was not the arthritis that prevented her from being as active as she wished but the side effects from the medicines she was taking for her hypertension. Karen did not pursue this.

The process of this interview betrayed Karen's secret: she had an underlying discomfort with pursuing medical data. Many things suggested this: her multiple questions in one breath, her abrupt shifts in topic, her flipping back and forth to her notes. Karen wanted to stay on surer ground and, for her, this meant the psychological history.

Just as some students can't sit still, others like Karen are afraid to take action, whether this action be directing a content-oriented medical history or, in later clinical years, performing medical and surgical procedures on their patients. Often this latter group of students, inhibited by medicine's technical side, hang back, rationalizing their failure to learn new procedures (such as a thoracentesis or lumbar puncture) on the basis that they're "going to be a psychiatrist."

This particular learning problem can be difficult to discern in introductory interviewing courses unless the preceptor is alert to it and unless such courses include a section on obtaining the medical history. Psychiatrist preceptors are more apt to miss this learning resistance than are teachers from other specialties. The best introductory interviewing courses are probably those that include some basic material on the content-directed medical history. Assisting students to shift from a receptive, empathic mode to a directive, content seeking mode will be discussed more fully in Part III. It suffices here to note that some medical students are afraid of medicine, and perhaps there is at least a grain of truth in the joke that psychiatrists are doctors who are afraid of blood. Often it is in the medical history taking portion of an interviewing course that preceptors can detect this learning difficulty and help the student take steps to overcome it.

Super-Student

Some people seem to have it all together, even in medical school. These are the students who always ask intelligent, cogent questions that impress the lecturer, though sometimes these questions seem to have been asked with just that motive in mind. Not only are they caught up in their course work, they've read a chapter ahead and can cite journal articles as well. They are the picture of confidence. When other students complain about the heavy workload or identity problems that medical school is creating, super-student seems perplexed and asks, "What's all the fuss about? I always leave aside 2½ hours at night to study and then go have fun—don't you?"

Clearly, the defense these students use is denial of anxiety through an illusion of omnipotence and absolute control. Such students often infuriate their peers, for whom life seems to be more of a struggle, yet it must be admitted that many such students do function very effectively, including in their clinical work with patients.

Nevertheless, if there is a chink in the armor, it tends to show up in their interactions with patients. Sometimes such students come across as calm, cool, and totally in the driver's seat. Yet, underneath, one senses an aloofness, a coldness, and a certain vague lack of empathy. They say all the right words, but the feelings don't seem to be there. It is as though their patients are objects to be analyzed and then forgotten. Such students can be a bit authoritarian; especially, they don't seem to have much patience for unruly emotions in their patients. This is understandable, in view of these students' wish to deny any similar potential in themselves. Superficially, such students may resemble the compulsive perfectionist, who sits at the bedside with his sheaf of notepads and outlines, scribbling madly. Yet, there is a critical difference. The compulsive perfectionist does convey to his patients a strong sense of commitment and concern. Sometimes, the super-student, rushing hurriedly past his patient's emotional expressions to get the "perfect" history, does not seem terribly concerned for his patients. It is almost as though the patient is there to aggrandize him. Despite a superficial finesse, such students often fail to become truly emotionally connected during their clinical work.

This is not to imply, of course, that all excellent, highly gifted students fall into this category. Yet there are those individuals who seem to display a subtle, unmistakable aloofness and egocentrism throughout their medical training. This trait is difficult to modify and educators are often left vaguely uneasy in their encounters with such students, feeling that despite their success (and such students often go on to achieve considerable prominence), "something is missing."

We could name other types of common learning difficulties—the excessively anxious student, the angry student, the self-effacing student. To lengthen the list unduly, however, would take us beyond the scope of this book. It is important, however, for students to recognize that individual style is a reality and that most of us tend to have our blind spots as well as our areas of strength. An important function of an interviewing course, therefore, includes helping the student to identify his style and to identify areas that he may avoid out of his own discomfort.

The Therapeutic Value of the Interview for the Patient

The ways in which a student's interview with his patient can be therapeutic have been elaborated elsewhere and need be reiterated only briefly here. The student's potential therapeutic contributions to his patient include the following.

Obtaining new data. Frequently the student's interview discloses important new data that contribute materially to that patient's clinical management and well being. Because students tend to be less constricted and content-bound in their approach to patients, they are often the first to uncover significant treatable depressions in their patients, important family problems, and socioeconomic difficulties. Many of these, once detected, are amenable to improvement. Students also, not infrequently, obtain additional valuable information about the patient's medical history.

The patient has a chance to share feelings. In the often harried pace of a typical medical ward, students can provide the patient with an important opportunity to discuss his feelings and concerns about being sick. This can substantially reduce the patient's anxiety. At the very least, providing a patient with this opportunity is humane. Beyond this, it is possible that a reduction in anxiety and depression can enhance a patient's sense of well being and speed his recovery. A less anxious, more hopeful patient will be better able to cooperate with his management in areas that range from physical therapy to medication compliance (in many studies patients have been shown to take their doctor's prescriptions as directed less than 50% of the time).

Furthermore, there is the hard to quantify yet widespread conviction of many clinicians that a sense of optimism and trust may directly affect the course of an illness. The converse has been better documented: patients with a history of depression or a recent loss have been shown to demonstrate a high rate of morbidity and mortality. Studies that demonstrate this include the work by Engel and Schmale on the "giving up-given up complex" and studies of morbidity and mortality rates among the recently bereaved. For instance, a widower is far more likely to die within 1 to 2 years after his spouse's death than is the general population. While the opposite is harder to prove, it seems plausible that a relationship that provides the patient with a sense of trust and well being can reduce the risk for morbidity and mortality.

Clarification of questions and problem areas. The student can often be instrumental in clarifying specific areas of patient concern and helping the patient to get something done about them. This help can range from such simple yet humane acts as Paul's procurement of a wig for Mrs. Clark in Chapter 1 to obtaining appropriate social service and pastoral or psychiatric intervention when these are indicated.

The student may be able to provide a patient with a meaningful doctor-patient relationship. It is ironic yet true that, in busy teaching hospitals and clinics, patients often become the property of an institution rather than the responsibility of an individual doctor. Clinic patients return week after week, year after year for chronic management of their problems. Their doctors change at least annually, often weekly. If these patients become acutely ill and require inpatient care, they are seldom treated by a doctor but rather by a "team." For the patient, this can be terrifying and incomprehensible. Often the only time they see their doctors is in the morning when a pack of five or more goes on rounds. In this situation, patients may have little notion of who their doctor really is—the intern, the junior resident, the senior resident, or the attending. Thus we often find the sad irony of a patient receiving the most sophisticated and advanced technological support that medicine can provide yet not being able to say who his doctor is.

The student can, if he wishes to commit himself, become a meaningful figure to such patients. Often the patients who most need the student in this way are those with the most depressing and frightening problems—the dying, the chronically ill, the depressed. These patients are the ones most apt to be shunted from one doctor to another, belonging to none. For a student to commit himself to such a patient, he needs to be willing to get involved in a relationship that may entail some risk of personal anxiety and pain.

This leads us to the final topic of this chapter.

Follow-up

In our experience, interviewing courses such as the one that we offer at the University of Colorado are increasingly common (though not universal) in medical schools. Most medical schools provide students with some opportunity to interview patients in a clinical setting during the first 2 years of their training and to discuss these experiences in a small group learning situation. Doubtless, the quality and substance of these courses vary greatly, but one thing we have been impressed with is the almost universal inattention to follow-up.

Most courses are structured around one-time exposures to patients. Afterwards the students group and discuss the interviews but seldom contemplate the possibility of following the patient over time. We believe this robs the student of a potentially meaningful, first hand experience of the doctor-patient relationship. Imagine if Paul had never gone back after that first interview to see Mrs. Clark.

This lack of follow-up has led to a legitimate complaint on the part of many students. They complain, in essence, that the interview situation is stilted because the students see the patient only once. This lends considerable fuel to the common student argument that the interview situation is a contrived one in which the student only pretends to be a doctor. These students have a point. Although the value of a single interview for a patient can be great, the patient is not permitted the opportunity to form a real relationship. This requires mutual commitment, gradual developing trust, and time.

Earlier in this book, we stated that a fundamental purpose of the small group learning situation is that of introducing the student to the experience of parallel process: the support and growth that the student experiences in his group can parallel a good doctor-patient relationship. Yet, in the final analysis, the student must have an opportunity to experience this relationship first hand with patients, not just in parallel.

For this reason, we strongly recommend that each student attempt to follow one of his patients over an extended period. Some medical schools do provide this opportunity. At Case Western Reserve University, for example, freshman medical students are introduced to a family at the beginning of prenatal care. The student then follows the family and child over the next 2 years. Other medical schools provide Continuity Clinics where students can follow patients over time. Such opportunities, however, should be more widespread.

Continuity experience of this kind should not be conducted without support and supervision, however. The doctor-patient relationship is like any very potent medicine; it has tremendous positive potential but also some hazardous side effects. While we commend Paul's valor and sense of personal responsibility to Mrs. Clark, it is too bad that he had to go it alone. Doing so poses potential emotional risks for the student and patient alike. At the very least, it deprives the student of a rich learning opportunity.

At some point in his training, each student needs to consolidate and integrate the intense experience of having a patient deeply involved with him. This is, after all, what he will be doing as a doctor for the rest of his life. Some students, from an understandable sense of anxiety, try to put off taking this step as long as they can. Frequently, we have heard students argue that they can't follow a patient "because I'm only a student. If I were an intern or resident, it would be different." But what is the ultimate effect of this? In our present educational system, students generally are never taught how to manage the doctor-patient relationship even though this will constitute the essence of what they are expected to do, and do skillfully, for the rest of their lives. At present, no phase of training provides adequately for this learning need. Introductory interviewing courses seem to be a logical place to begin to introduce students to this aspect of patient management.

Ideally, the student should arrange to develop a follow-up relationship with at least one patient whom he interviews during the course of a year. This patient should be selected with some care by the preceptor and course directors with consideration for the learning needs of the student and the therapeutic needs of the patient being paramount. Finally, supervision and teaching should be provided to the student during the period that he follows his patient.

References

Davis, M: Variations in compliance with doctor's orders: Analysis of congruence between survey responses and results of empirical investigations. *J. Med. Educ., 41:*1037, 1966.

Engel, G. L.: A life setting conducive to illness: The giving up-given up complex. *Ann. Intern. Med., 69:*293, 1968.

Ford, A. B., Liske, R. E., Ort, R. S., and Denton, J. C.: *The Doctor's Perspective: Physicians View Their Patients and Practice.* The Press of Case Western Reserve University, Cleveland, Ohio, 1967.

Friedman, R. C.: Stress, sleep and the house officer. *Continuing Medical Education Newsletter, V:*22, 1974.

Pardes, H.: The discussion group experience in the teaching of human behavior. In *Understanding Human Behavior in Health and Illness,* edited by Richard C. Simons and Herbert Pardes. Williams & Wilkins, Baltimore, 1977.

Schmale, A. H., and Engel, G. L.: The giving up-given up complex illustrated on film. *Arch. Gen. Psychiatry., 17:*135, 1967.

part III

THE
MEDICAL
HISTORY

chapter 8

COMPONENTS OF THE MEDICAL HISTORY

COMMON PROBLEMS IN HISTORY TAKING

Although the primary focus of this chapter is on the components of the
medical history, students are so routinely stymied by certain common
problems when they begin to obtain medical histories that some discussion
of these problems seems pertinent at the outset.

Shifting Gears

Students usually find the process of shifting gears with a patient from an
empathic, open-ended stance to a content-directed, probing, history-seeking
stance difficult. They feel awkward and often frustrated that they cannot
seem to do so in a smooth and synchronous way. Especially at the outset, it
seems extremely difficult to form a close alliance with a patient, develop an
atmosphere of empathy and rapport, achieve an understanding of the
patient's process communications, and then, on top of all this, also probe in
detail the exact nature, duration, and quality of a patient's symptoms. We
will discuss some effective approaches in Chapter 9. It suffices here to say
that this ability to shift gears *is* difficult to achieve and remains a challenge
even for experienced clinicians.

Problems of Time and Setting

In an ideal clinical situation, it is important to have latitude in how one
plans his time. Prior to sitting down with any new patient to obtain a medical
history, an experienced and unharried clinician will try to predict how much
time he needs to spend with that patient, judge what is the best time to
interview the patient, and consider the possible need for future interviews.
Patients may fatigue easily, especially if hospitalized, and may need to
interrupt an interview before it is finished. A patient's emotional response to

163

material that comes up during an interview may occasionally require that certain other aspects of information gathering be postponed. It is frustrating to have expectations of obtaining a complete interview in one sitting only to be interrupted by the patient's being called to x-ray or by a consultant's visit. It helps, therefore, to be realistic about time and to approach every new patient with a certain degree of anticipation that, in fact, everything may not go exactly according to schedule. Schwartz emphasizes the value of multiple meetings. He has observed that a period between interviews often permits both patient and physician to consolidate their thinking and sharpen their focus about the current medical problem.

Unfortunately, no such ideal state exists in the training centers where medical students are most likely to be interviewing their first patients. Typically, students will receive the bulk of their training in overcrowded, understaffed public clinics, university and city hospital teaching wards, and VA hospitals. The ambience in these settings falls far short of the quiet, leather-bound study image that we all dreamed of when watching *Marcus Welby*. Instead, the student is likely to find his first clinical contacts occurring on busy wards where there may be four or more patients to a room, televisions blaring, people tromping in and out during the interview, and, generally, a certain unnerving level of chronic institutional chaos. Most medical personnel can and do adapt to such environments over time or at least become able to tolerate them. But the beginning student often finds this sort of undercurrent especially irksome because he is already concentrating hard on mastering the task at hand and does not welcome any distractions. The hazard in all of this is that students sometimes experience excessive frustration and develop a chronic cynicism that invariably gets transmitted to the patient. Patients who are treated in these settings are already quite vulnerable to this frustration because they are far from immune to the same distractions and tensions that the student experiences. It is important, therefore, to remember that the interview does not represent an ideal situation for the patient either, who is already touchy about "accepting charity" on a public ward. In most instances, a good doctor-patient relationship can transcend these frustrations. In the beginning, the student will have to be prepared for them—even resigned to them.

Problems with the Patient Population

As we will make clearer in Chapter 9, a very important clinical skill is the capacity to differentiate between subjective and objective data. Ideally, the medical interview is that section of a patient's evaluation during which the clinician tunes in most intensively to the patient's subjective experience of illness. As a physician, you will want to know how symptoms started, how they evolved, and how the patient felt as they evolved. During the course of your professional practice, you will treat a patient who has in many instances already been evaluated and treated by other doctors. You will want to know, of course, how they came to their conclusions about your patient. Still, each new medical interview should be viewed as an opportunity to start afresh—to listen to a story that may well have been told before but to listen through your own ears for the first time. This is, at the very least, alliance building. Not infrequently, a new clinician, even one in a long line of clinicians, will hear something new or else will put the same story together in a new way that enhances the patient's future management and care.

Obviously, the ability to produce a clear, pertinent, intelligible history depends on the verbal skills of the patient as well as on the interviewing skills of the clinician. Thus, ideal qualities in a patient whom a beginning student might be interviewing would include intelligence, the ability to be articulate, and organization in thinking. In addition, a fairly straightforward medical problem can be especially valuable for students at the beginning of training when they are trying to perfect their history taking. Patients with certain straightforward syndromes that present classically can make learning interviewing much easier. This would be the ideal.

Here, though, is the reality: the student will interview patients who have not only been treated by a long succession of doctors in the past but who are now being treated by two or three doctors at once, in a clinic or teaching hospital setting. The odds are great that these patients will be socioeconomically and educationally deprived. They may well be cynical and angry about the treatment they have received, not only at the hands of the health care establishment, but indeed at the hands of life. They will seldom be able to articulate their history in a clear and concise manner. Furthermore, their medical histories are apt to be complex—long litanies of chronic illnesses and treatment regimens, complicated side effects, and muddled pharmacologic interactions. The student, as a beginning interviewer, is apt to feel a bit like someone who has signed up for a course in beginning mountaineering and then is handed a pair of snowshoes and told to go climb Mt. McKinley.

Beyond this, such patients, as historians, will not describe the evolution of their illness as they experienced it. Rather, they will give a long description of secondary and tertiary inferences made by other clinicians during the course of their management. "Well, doctor, I'm here because of what they think is Wegener's Granulomatosis. The first doctor in Memorial thought it was just pneumonia but then this other expert came in and he did some kidney tests, and then another expert came in and he did a biopsy and they said, 'Yep, sure, it's Wegener's Granulomatosis, alright.' So they sent me over here to the University. Doctor Hotler says he thinks it's Wegener's Granulomatosis, but he wants to do some more tests and he thinks it might be a rare subtype that he says he's written about in a journal."

Such frequent complications do not provide the student with the most effective material to easily learn history taking at the outset of his training. Material of this kind can come only from a patient who has applied for treatment relatively recently—and for a relatively straightforward problem. Such patients exist, but students seldom see them. They are seen instead by private practitioners in the community. In the topsy-turvy world of American medicine, the student must reconcile himself to seeing the most complex and confusing patients from the outset. It helps, however, to remember that a great service may be done for these patients when students and house staff succeed in obtaining an empathic, thorough history, which ultimately formulates such patients' problems accurately and comprehensively.

Erroneous Expectations of How the Medical History Unfolds

Of all the types of disenchantment that a student is apt to feel as he begins to obtain medical histories, none is more startling than the difference between the way a patient (even an organized patient) tells his story and the way one reads about it in textbooks. During the course of their education, students have come to expect that ideas should unfold in a rational, understandable sequence of steps. The fact that this ideal is rarely attained, even in education, is attested to by the massive appreciation that students feel for the occasional lecturer who actually presents his material in an organized, coherent way. Nevertheless, the *expectation* that is imbued in the student from the outset is that a disease has a logical progression and unfolds according to certain principles and rules. When one reads a textbook of medicine, one reads about a "classic" illness, with "classical" stages, symptoms, and progression. In reality, diseases, even the simplest of them, are rarely so classical.

Moreover, patients are not apt to present their experience of illness in such a logical and orderly fashion. The concerns each patient expresses most prominently will vary. One may be more concerned about his car being parked in a tow-away zone in front of the ER than he is with how long he has had chest pain. Another will focus on symptoms that, to him, are highly distressing but to the clinician may be distracting asides. An elderly woman with a congestive heart failure may seem more concerned about constipation than she is with ankle edema, at least on the surface. Such patients are not "bad" patients; they are *typical*.

The student must learn quickly that the goal of the medical history is to obtain the most lucid, chronologically exact, historically pertinent depiction possible of a patient's illness. His goal, furthermore, should be to write this down, report it to colleagues, and think about it in an equally cognizant and organized manner. The actual *process* of obtaining a medical history, however, will involve vastly different skills.

Like all other patient communications, the medical history too will be communicated largely in process. The order in which a patient chooses to bring up symptoms will be important. Areas of obscurity will be as pertinent as areas of clarity. What a patient leaves out may be critical. To begin to develop skills in listening to the medical history as it unfolds in process is difficult; it represents a lifelong challenge. We will discuss this further in Chapter 9. Here, it is most important to state that many clinicians at all levels of experience—especially those who do not understand that a patient's history unfolds as process—are apt to become put-out and frustrated with many patients, to the detriment of the process unfolding. These clinicians will evince a hurry-up attitude, interrupting the patient and urging him to get on to what the clinician regards as "important." Such a clinician's face will often bear an unmistakable expression of annoyance as he taps his foot and begrudgingly waits for the patient to finish his next sentence so that he can get on with obtaining the "important information." Such an attitude is often based on the physician's underlying fantasy that patients can and should be able to present their diseases in the same logical sequence that clinicians ultimately think about them. Nothing could be further from the truth! Clinicians who fail to appreciate this distinction not only create poor alliances with their patients but often obtain data that are faulty and inaccurate as a result.

THE COMPONENTS

Recording data about each patient in the following format has become standard medical practice; this format is also used routinely in presenting cases to colleagues.
1. Identifying Data
2. Informant
3. Chief Complaint
4. Present Illness
5. Past History
6. Family History
7. Review of Systems
8. Social History/Patient Profile

In a patient's chart, these data are followed by the report of the physical examination. Thus, when the student learns these components of the medical history, he is not learning our schema in particular but one that is universally adhered to and applied. How the student actually obtains these data, however, is subject to great variability; plans of attack differ considerably among clinicians. The approach that we advocate will be explicated in Chapter 9.

Identifying Data

Identifying data are expressed in a concise, one-sentence summary. They include the patient's name, age, race, marital status, and occupation and why the patient has come—the reason for the medical work-up. Occasionally this section may be expanded slightly; for instance, neurologists often include an indication of right- or left-handedness under identifying data, and some clinicians appropriately throw in a fact that is not classically part of the identifying data but that may be of special importance. Identifying data, however, should be terse. Thus, one might say: "This is the first hospital admission for Mr. Robert W. Johnson, a 39-year-old white married man, employed as a licensed practical nurse at a local metropolitan hospital, admitted now for evaluation of chest pain and fever." One might expand on this slightly, but only to a minimal degree. Thus, one might add that Mr. Johnson is the father of three children or that he is currently working as an LPN while he goes to nursing school to obtain an RN degree. Identifying data are not the place for much embellishment, however.

The purposes of identifying data are to tell anyone who refers to the record who the patient is, to lock a memory of the patient in the clinician's mind, and to give a brief thumbnail sketch of certain very pertinent pieces of historical data that consistently have a great deal to say about the type of patient one is dealing with and the reason for the medical evaluation.

Telling People Who the Patient Is

In a classic example of black humor, the contemporary film *Hospital* depicts a series of mishaps that occur because patients are misidentified: beds get swapped, the wrong patient gets operated on, etc. While the movie's effect is sardonic and comical, mishaps do occur in reality. One mundane, yet absolutely critical purpose for identifying data is the prevention of such mix-ups.

Locking The Patient Into the Clinician's Mind

An important way in which we all develop increasing clinical competence is by seeing a variety of pathology, dysfunction, and disease in a wide range of patients. Reading about diseases and dysfunctions from textbooks and journals can be helpful; but without the experience of seeing a specific person with a specific syndrome, our recall tends to be poor. Identifying data are one small but important way that a clinician has of associating the disease pathology that he is studying with people he specifically remembers.

The Diagnostic Value of Identifying Data

A great deal of important information about a patient can be contained in a terse biographical sketch. For instance, a 39-year-old man with no permanent address, no phone, single, and unemployed is strikingly different from a 39-year-old married LPN who is studying for an RN degree. They will have had many different influences on their lives that have molded them in very important ways. Physiologically, too, they are different, being exposed to and prone to different illnesses and dysfunctions. Should they contract the same disease, furthermore, their physiologic response may well be markedly different.

Presenting the Patient As a Person With a Problem

Whether by wisdom or accident, placing the identifying data first in a medical history says this is a person before he is a disease, and no matter how fascinating or urgent his illness is, his existence as a human being comes first. Beyond this, when a physician presents his patient to a colleague, the identifying data serve as a frame of reference for the case presentation as a whole. This frame of reference, whether written or verbal, prepares the listener (often an attending with wide clinical experience) to expect that certain data will emerge in the presentation that follows. The listener, having been properly introduced, will be able to listen to the case in a far more directed and sentient manner. This obviously makes more sense than presenting the case as a mystery story of sorts with the "answer" at the end. In a real sense, at the time the identifying data are formulated in the student's mind, the entire initial work-up should be largely complete; the distillation of key data from this work-up then forms the appropriate elements of the identifying data—an *introduction* to the remainder of the work-up. It directs attention to what will follow. Consistently excellent examples of brief statements that answer the question, "Why was the patient seen now?" occur in the Case Records of the Massachusetts General Hospital that appears as a regular feature in the *New England Journal of Medicine*. Two examples follow:

1. A 5 y/o boy was admitted to the hospital because of hyperinflation of the upper lobe of the left lung.
2. A 70 y/o man was admitted to the hospital because of back pain.

Combining the personal identity of the patient with a simple statement about the reason for admission (or presentation in the outpatient clinic) is, in our opinion, the best opening for a medical history: Thus;

This is the 10th Denver General Hospital admission for this 59 y/o single white male postal worker admitted for evaluation of recurrent ascites.

Or

Mary Elkins is a 49 y/o black married female who presented to medical clinic for evaluation of constant (bitemporal) headaches.

As the reader will see, a comparison of the identifying data (including the reason for the evaluation) with the patient's chief complaint can often give us immediate insight into any gaps between the medical reason for the work-up and the patient's concept of what he needs help with. This gap can and must be dealt with. Denial and lack of information are the two most common reasons for such a gap, though obviously many others are possible. Lack of information is easily corrected. Denial, as we discussed in Chapter 4, is a more complex patient reaction that requires an individually tailored response based on the needs, apprehensions, and developmental state of the patient. One does not always attack denial in a frontal assault like Don Quixote plunging at a windmill. Usually, with understanding from the physician, patients will discover the "truth" in graduated steps, at their own appropriate pace.

Informant

Usually this is the patient but sometimes may be a family member or friend. This should be stated clearly. In addition, some clinicians use this section of the medical history to assess the patient's reliability as a historian. Thus, "The history was given by the patient, who is regarded as a reliable informant." Or, "History by neighbor, patient comatose."

Chief Complaint

This is the *patient's* statement of the reason he has come to see you now (as opposed to the identifying data, which is *your interpretation* of why he has come now). Usually, it should be one sentence, almost never more than two. It should reflect the most critical priority in the patient's mind at the time you are interviewing him. When possible, it should be presented in the patient's own words, placed in quotations, such as "I've been coughing a lot and yesterday I started to get a fever." The chief complaint is the patient's statement and does not necessarily reflect the clinician's sense of what is most important, except when patient and clinician happen to agree. To take one example, a 30-year-old chronic schizophrenic man was brought to our emergency room not long ago because he had fallen to the sidewalk while walking his dog and gone into convulsions. The patient was bewildered and disoriented. He screamed, "Don't touch me! Don't touch me! You're agents of Satan!" The proper chief complaint here might read "Don't touch me! Don't touch me! You're agents of Satan!" Or it might be toned down (less preferable) to a statement such as "The patient can give no specific chief complaint, stating only that he has been brought against his will and that the hospital staff are agents of Satan." The gap between the clinician's understanding of the problem and the patient's understanding is obviously great in this example. The patient here does not make any mention of the critical importance of his convulsions. However this latter fact belongs in the identifying data, not in the chief complaint. The chief complaint is a statement that most accurately represents, in one sentence, the pressing concern on the patient's mind. Record it accurately and simply; don't embellish or editorialize on it.

Present Illness

A student will frequently hear during his training that the medical history contains the most important data concerning a patient's illness—more important than the physical examination, the laboratory values, the arteriography, or the computerized tomography scan. As is true of any principle, the importance of this statement can become exaggerated, but often the medical history *is* crucial. Within the medical history, it is the history of present illness that is usually most important. Obtaining a precise, well organized account of present illness is also the most difficult part of the medical history. We feel so strongly about both the importance and difficulty of the history of present illness in our own course that we encourage students and preceptors to focus on it for as long as need be. We feel that, once a student has begun to master this element, he can pick up the other parts of the history with much greater ease.

Patients do not usually present their story in a logical, chronological sequence. They present it in bits and pieces, fits and starts, as they interpret their distress through a prism of fear, pain, life experiences, and personal priorities. The typical patient provides some data about the present problem, recounts an aside about something that happened to one of his parents, follows with a question, and then adds some seemingly unrelated information from the past. The clinician's task is no small one. He must be able to listen receptively and creatively to the rhythm, timing, and sequence of the patient's own account—the process—while simultaneously attempting to organize this account into a coherent system of data that pertains to the patient's present illness and its manifestations. A great deal of discretion, clinical experience, and judgment go into deciding how long to let a patient follow his own associations and when to step in and become more focused and directive. This will be discussed further in Chapter 9.

Where Does The Present Illness Begin?

The present illness begins with what brings the patient to you *now*. Sometimes this is clearcut. Often it is not. In the case of a previously healthy person who suddenly develops acute symptoms, the onset of present illness is straightforward. Frequently, however patients present with a new development in a chronic disease. For example, a patient with diabetes may have a very complicated medical history. He may come to you now because he has noticed a recent worsening of vision in his right eye. In this case, the present illness begins with the eye problem. Thus, the beginning of a present illness for such a patient might read: "This 45-year-old man, with a chronic, complex medical history related to juvenile onset *diabetes mellitus*, presents with a 2-week history of visual difficulties in his right eye..."

This principle is not foolproof, however. A patient may come to you with a 6-month history of progressive rheumatoid arthritis. He is applying for care now because the joints in his fingers are hurting especially badly. Does the present illness begin with pain in the fingers, which got worse this morning? Or does it begin with the onset of arthritic symptoms a few months ago? Probably, in this case, the present illness still begins with the finger pain from this morning; but one can quickly see that there are many possible shades of gray. Sometimes, the point at which to start the account of present illness is discretionary and based on the clinician's experience.

As a general rule, we recommend that the first paragraph of the history of present illness begin with the most immediate complaint in time. With the exception of those patients who are unable to articulate it clearly, the chief complaint usually provides the most reliable clue.

The question then arises, where does one put pertinent recent information clearly related to the present illness that preceded the most current problem? Does the clinician include this information in the past history only or also include it in the present illness? We recommend, in general, that pertinent symptoms which are probably related to the current problem be entered in subsequent paragraphs of the present illness. Thus, to take the case of the man with eye problems related to his diabetes, the first paragraph of the present illness should be devoted to developing a detailed description of the most immediate problem—the eye problem—according to parameters to be described below. After this has been done, the clinician may begin a new paragraph, still continuing the present illness, which traces the current disease in a more general way from its origins to the present. Thus, the second paragraph of this patient's present illness might begin: "Mr. Goodrich was first diagnosed as having diabetes mellitus at age 7, at which time a family physician noted the classic onset of urinary frequency, thirst, and hunger accompanied by weight loss. He was well controlled on daily subcutaneous doses of semilente insulin until his mid-20s, when he began to experience renal and, later, cardiac complications secondary to his diabetes. Recurrent problems, especially with advancing renal failure, have necessitated numerous admissions to the hospital over the years. Currently, this patient's renal status appears to be well controlled, but for the last year he has complained for the first time of increasing visual difficulties, primarily in his right eye..."

The reader should note three things about developing the present illness in this way. First, the earlier history of the same disease should be presented in more general fashion, but how general is still a matter that requires clinical discretion; it often depends on the experience and, to an extent, the tastes of the individual clinician. Second, the astute reader will notice that the second paragraph mixes subjective and objective data somewhat unclearly. Strictly speaking, the present illness should be carefully developed according to the patient's subjective experience of the illness. Giving an overview increases the likelihood of bringing in surmises about what has been objective data in the past. Here, for instance, did the cardiac and renal problems referred to get reported in those words by the patient? Did the clinician deduce from the patient's general description that they were cardiac and renal? Or does the clinician know this from reviewing the patient's chart? We do not know. Clearly, there is potential here for ambiguity. However, we feel that the logic of including earlier details of a disease in overview outweights this risk, if the clinician is aware of what he is doing. Third, and most important, it is chancy sometimes to assume that a new problem is automatically related to an older disease. For example, this patient could be developing glaucoma or blindness due to some other cause. The clinician must be very careful about jumping to conclusions, a skill that obviously develops over time but fools all of us periodically. If a student is in significant doubt about whether a current symptom relates to a previous disease, it is wisest to restrict the present illness to the current difficulty and then elaborate the history of the chronic disease under the past history.

What about the patient who presents with two or three complaints? To give one example, a 25-year-old woman presented in our emergency room because of severe chest pain. However, she also noted that in the last few months she had had frequent skin rashes and ulcerations on the tips of her toes and sometimes stabbing pain in her knees and elbows. From these symptoms alone, it is hard to tell whether the patient has several different problems or one related problem. An ancient, venerated rule in medicine— indeed a very reliable one—is the law of parsimony, which states that one attempts to explain as many symptoms as possible on the basis of as few underlying diseases as possible. This is not always so simple, however, especially early in the course of certain illnesses. In this case, the law of parsimony did indeed apply. This woman was suffering from systemic lupus erythematosis, a disease involving many organ systems, which can present in this way. To expect a clinician to figure this out, however, on the basis of the presenting symptoms alone, would be wrong. In fact it would represent sloppy clinical thinking, because a number of other diseases could cause this same picture. In situations where the patient's present illness seems to consist of several unrelated, or questionably related, symptoms, each should be developed separately in a separate paragraph of the present illness. Again, the first paragraph should begin with the most immediate problem, which in this patient's case was chest pain. Then, in subsequent paragraphs, the clinician can develop the other symptoms: "This woman has also complained of the onset of joint pain, occurring in different joints, for the last three months . . ."

One can see many areas of potential uncertainty. A general principle is, start with what brought the patient to you *now*.

The Seven Dimensions of the Present Illness

Morgan and Engel have proposed that the clinician use seven dimensions as a framework for clarifying the present illness: chronology, bodily location, quality, quantity, setting, aggravating or alleviating factors, and associated manifestations. These seven parameters can serve as an invaluable guide to the beginning clinician in organizing a description of the present illness. Furthermore, the clinician who has mastered their use can apply these same parameters to any symptoms of illness uncovered in the medical history. While we generally recommend against memorization and rote learning in this book, if the student were to memorize one thing, it should be these seven dimensions. They do have limitations for they do not describe all diseases equally well. Some diseases do not manifest in all seven dimensions; others have symptoms that are not fully encompassed by these categories. By and large, however, their use in history taking is very reliable.

Chronology. Of the seven dimensions, chronology is the most important. Dates and times when symptoms first began are consistently the most reliable descriptors with which to develop the present illness. If you observe good clinicians obtaining a present illness, you will see great variability in their styles of questioning. Invariably, however, you will see frequent, indeed almost monotonous, references to time of onset. "So when did that begin again?" "So as I understand it, you first noted the swelling in your knee 2 weeks ago." "So let me go over that again—2 weeks ago you noticed swelling in your knee, and then it was 3 days after that that the rash first appeared." It is impossible to overstate the importance of scrupulous attention to detail in dating of the onset of symptoms.

There are two prevailing styles for recording these data. Some clinicians date symptoms by saying, "*Three weeks prior to admission* the patient developed a high fever. *Two weeks prior to admission* he began to experience a severe cough and shortness of breath. *One day prior to admission*, while rising from the bed, he became faint and fell to the floor, losing consciousness." The advantage to such a system of recording is its simplicity. A clinician reading a chart 6 weeks into a patient's admission may occasionally get confused by calendar dates and times. He will have to thumb through the chart for the date of admission and then do some mental arithmetic to organize his time framework. We believe that the advantages of this system, however, are outweighed by the disadvantages. We recommend using calendar dates and times in recording, as well as obtaining, the present illness. In order to make the task of "translating" intervals simpler for future clinicians, we recommend this: immediately under the heading of the present illness put a calendar date, e.g., "recorded at 3:01 p.m., November 21, 1979." In this way, a clinician reading the chart years later can refer to this date to organize his time frame. The major advantage to using precise dates and times is their inherent service to exactness.

Patients are notoriously inaccurate about dates. "About 3 weeks ago" is not good enough. It must be nailed down. "Do you remember the day of the week?" If the patient doesn't know, "How many days after the weekend was it? If you don't remember the time, was it morning or afternoon; before or after lunch?" The importance of this attention to detail is critical. No clinician should begin his relationship with a patient by demanding such precision of detail; but he must begin to gradually narrow down a period of time and focus on precise dates and times.

It is especially important to establish the onset of the first symptoms. Patients often minimize early prodromal symptoms that seem unimportant to them but which are very critical diagnostically. A good rule of thumb is, always try to establish the last time when the patient felt in his usual state of health. Sometimes, when the patient has trouble with dates, anchoring the history to holidays and events can help. "Was that before or after the Christmas holidays? After Christmas, but before New Year's?" This kind of specificity is also very valuable because it often prods the patient into suddenly "remembering" that he was feeling "a bit beat" 2 weeks before the swelling in his knee.

When patients *do* remember dates exactly, it is important to inquire about related events. Usually they will be important. Morgan and Engel give the example of a patient who said, without hesitation, that his first episode of chest pain occurred at 7:15 p.m., March 3, 1967. It turned out that he remembered the date exactly because he had received word that day that his son had been injured in an auto accident. He remembered the precise time because he was watching the evening news on TV when the pain began.

Bodily Location. Patients generally refer to bodily location in lay terms, rather than technical ones, and broadly rather than specifically—"headache," "stomach ache," "backache." It is up to the clinician to localize this more precisely. Sometimes it is helpful to get the patient to point. "Can you point your finger to exactly where on your belly it hurts the most?" Questions related to depth are useful, since patients often can tell, in a general way, whether the pain feels on the surface of their body or deep. *Radiation* is an essential dimension to explore. Where does the pain go? Through to the back? Down into the left arm? Up to the jaw?

Quality. Begin generally by asking the patient what the pain is like. If he begins with very vague terms, it is often useful to ask him to relate it to some similar pain he has experienced. Sometimes, however, it is necessary for the clinician to ask leading questions. Was the pain sharp or dull? Constant or intermittent? Throbbing or stabbing? Giving the patient a choice reduces the likelihood of "leading the witness," but the less articulate a patient is, the more likely will the physician be to offer the patient his own adjectives from which to choose.

Quantity. Important questions related to quantity include frequency, size, volume, and number. "How many times did you vomit?" " How much did you vomit?" Again, it is important to be specific. "Do you think it was six or eight times, or more like three or four?" If the patient says he vomited "a lot," what did that mean? "Would it fill a 6-ounce paper cup?" Some symptoms are so emotionally charged for a patient that specificity is difficult to obtain. Bleeding is an example. A patient may say that he's been coughing up "a lot of blood" when it turns out to be less than a teaspoon. The intensity of the symptoms, in terms of pain or degree of impairment, can sometimes be ascertained by asking a patient to compare it to something similar. "What was the worst pain you've ever had?" "If, on a scale of 1 to 10, that was a 10, how bad is this pain?"

The degree of functional impairment is best quantified by getting specific details about what a patient can do. If a patient has previously been able to sew for 2 hours every afternoon before her arthritis became too painful, how long can she sew now—an hour? Only a few minutes? Not at all?

Setting. A student will have a much easier time establishing the setting in which the patient's illness has developed if he has already developed a good rapport and communicated his interest in the whole person, not just in his symptoms. Patients who receive such attention frequently volunteer the setting in which their symptoms occur—"Often I find it's worse late at night. It's not just the time of day—though I *do* think the stiffness gets worse then—but it's hard—at night, when you're all alone, nothing to think about but the kids, and they're all grown."

Another reason for inquiring about setting is its relationship to certain illnesses. The frenzy of an accountant's office at tax preparation time is obviously relevant when a CPA comes in with burning epigastric pain. A history of exposure to certain toxins, as seen in employees of an asbestos factory or coal mine, gives important clues to possible causes of a pulmonary complaint. For someone who has just returned from Mexico with diarrhea, setting is of great significance.

Aggravating or Alleviating Factors. What makes the symptoms better or worse? Did exercise make the chest pain increase? Did the knee pain go away after the morning jog or did it get worse? Did milk help relieve the indigestion? Or did food make it worse?

Associated Manifestations. Once a patient has recounted the other six dimensions of his illness, it is always useful to probe for anything else that the patient has noticed associated with the symptoms, however seemingly trivial to him. Your ability to elicit data in this dimension will depend on your clinical experience and knowledge of pathophysiology. A clinician who is familiar with systemic lupus erythematosis, for example, is much more likely to ask a young woman with joint pain about rashes and unexplained fever. Even the beginning clinician, however, can ask for "anything else— anything at all that you remember?" Dr. Reiser's illness, described in Chapter 3, underscores the importance of eliciting a history of associated manifestations. Here, the association was very subtle; but, if a clinician had asked much earlier—"Did you have any other symptoms or illnesses, anything at all in the past few weeks?"—the trivial skin cyst and casually prescribed antibiotic that led to the diagnosis of colitis might have been remembered.

With each of these seven parameters of illness, the student's skill, experience, and knowledge of pathophysiology will be important. Often, beginning students feel needless but understandable exasperation and discouragement when they do not know what questions to ask. There *are* limitations based on the student's level of training. Of all the seven parameters, chronology requires the least specific knowledge of pathophysiology and is also the most important. Questions that pertain to quantity and quality also depend more on creativity and attention to detail than on sophisticated clinical knowledge. A great deal of the patient's present illness can be described by these parameters alone. When this description can be enhanced by descriptors in the other parameters, this is all for the better, but even the beginning student can aspire to obtaining a careful chronological account of his patient's present illness.

Finally, a careful present illness includes *pertinent negatives* as well as positive symptoms. A patient, for instance, who comes in with chest pain that is not aggravated by exercise or exertion is telling the clinician something very important by ruling out what he does *not* have. Here again, however, beginning clinicians must tolerate the constraints imposed by their level of clinical experience. A student who has not yet learned about angina pectoris may have no way of knowing why a negative history for exercise intolerance is an important finding. The importance of negative findings will also be discussed further in Chapter 9.

Past History

Past history includes a review of: (1) immunizations, (2) childhood and adult illnesses, (3) significant injuries, (4) surgical procedures, (5) hospitalizations, (6) present medications, and (7) drug sensitivities.

Most of the items recorded in a past history should be included to provide important historical information but generally should not be directly pertinent to the present illness. If the clinician has discerned a relationship between a past event and the present problem, this should be recorded in a later paragraph of the present illness, as described above. Obviously, at times, a clinician will not be sure of the significance of a past event and may record something in the past history that *does* relate to the present. A very simple example would be a patient who presents with symptoms of congestive heart failure secondary to mitral stenosis. A clinician who is not familiar with the close correlation between rheumatic fever in childhood and later mitral stenosis might well record a history of rheumatic fever in the past history, whereas a more experienced clinician would mention this fact as the past history of the present illness, *entered* under the present illness.

The student who has mastered the seven dimensions of the present illness will be able to apply them to illnesses from the past as well, if this is indicated. Generally, however, the past history should be brief and to the point.

Family History

The family history is an important part of the patient's medical history. It should include the age and health of the parents, or their age at death and the cause of death. The age and health, or cause of death, of siblings should also be enumerated. In some cases, a more detailed family tree may be important. For example, in certain kinds of depression, there is good evidence that the illness can be transmitted over several generations, and a family history is therefore especially important. Clinician experience is important in this section of the history. With time, the physician learns which diseases are transmitted in a familial pattern and which are therefore most relevant to ask about. A minimum family history consists of knowing the state of health of the parents and siblings. When possible, paternal and maternal grandparents should be included, as well as the patient's children. Some students like to do this section of the history in diagrammatic form.

The student should be prepared for a patient's emotional reactions during the recounting of the family history. This seemingly routine phase of the medical interview is, in fact, centered on highly charged emotional issues— is a parent still alive?. If not, how did he die? Has a patient lost a child through accident or disease? Has a brother been psychiatrically commited? The student should be observant during this phase of the history and be prepared to pause and encourage the patient's thoughts and feelings rather than to brusquely hurry on to the next question.

Review of Systems

The review of systems is the clinician's final historical cross-check. After a thorough history of present illness and past history, the clinician will usually encounter no surprises during the review of the systems. This is a final scanning inventory designed to uncover any overlooked problems in the major organ systems. Many surveys have been devised. In practice, clinicians vary greatly in the depth and detail of their own reviews of systems. Initially, it is impossible for students to memorize the list of questions necessary for an adequate review of systems. For this purpose, we have developed an appendix to which the student can refer when obtaining a review of systems. There is nothing wrong with referring to this inventory with the book open during this phase of the interview.

Students will quickly become acquainted with the phenomenon of the "positive historian." This is the patient who answers "yes" to one question after another. Usually such patients are anxious about their illness and may be anxious about their health in general. A student can feel overwhelmed by the mass of positive data that suddenly spills out. What does he do with all this new information? How deeply should he explore each positive finding? Here again, experience helps. If the clinician has obtained a good history, the organ system review should be relatively noncontributory. Platt and McMath have found that many doctors have problems with patients who are positive historians. They suggest a technique for "emptying" the review of systems. They propose that this be done by asking questions, such as the following, after completing the history: "What other sorts of problems have you been having lately?" "How are you otherwise?" "What else is bothering you?" As they point out, these problems may be medical, social, psychological, or financial. If this step is taken, the review of systems should be largely negative. If the clinician still finds the review of systems highly positive, he is most likely dealing with someone who is frightened or in some other way deeply preoccupied with his state of health and physical functioning. This finding, in turn, will require attention and follow-up; but usually it will involve an attempt to understand the patient's underlying concerns rather than chasing one red herring after another in the medical work-up.

Social History/Patient Profile

Nowhere in the standard medical history is there more confusion, amounting at times to nonsense, than in the so-called social history. The typical social history at a busy city hospital is apt to be one line: "Smokes 2 ppd. Etoh mod." This sort of parody of the social history tells us absolutely nothing of importance about the patient as a person. Yet, how far to the other extreme should one go? The clinician cannot, and obviously should not, write a biography that rambles on for pages about every patient's life. We suggest a compromise: a paragraph or two (at the most) that attempts to convey the essence of this patient as a person. Topics might include: (1) birth place, (2) occupation, (3) education, (4) usual daily activities, (5) housing, (6) financial status, (7) availability of family and friends, and (8) risk habits (including use of prescribed and nonprescribed drugs, alcohol use, smoking habits, etc.). Other topics may occur to the student as well.

This should not be done as a list. Being able to condense one's understanding of a patient and to articulate it in a concise, yet lively manner is an important clinical skill. With some practice, the student should be able to develop his ability to paint a brief but meaningful picture of his patients. For example,

> The patient was born in West Virginia and educated through the 11th grade. He was raised by his grandmother due to his parents' separation when he was 3 and mother's death in an auto accident 1 year later. At age 8, he moved with his grandmother and his 2 siblings to Cleveland where he remained for most of his adult life. After high school he worked as a "shake-out man" in a foundry for 12 years, then held odd jobs for 5 years. For the past 8 years he has driven a truck until forced to quit and seek disability due to an on-the-job injury which has caused chronic low back pain. He has been married twice, the first time ending in divorce after 15 years, the second, his current marriage, now in its 14th year. He has 4 grown children and lives in his own 3 bedroom home with his wife, her sister and her 3 small children. He has a 24 pack-year smoking history and is a social drinker. A typical day begins at 7:30 a.m. when he arises, eats breakfast, and goes to physical therapy at a local clinic. He skips lunch, naps in the afternoon and spends the rest of the day laying on the couch watching TV. He occasionally helps with dinner (he enjoys cooking) and watches more TV after dinner until he retires at about 10:30. He eats protein and fresh vegetables daily, but lacks grain and dairy products regularly in his diet. Hobbies include stamp collecting and working in his yard, neither of which he can do because of his back problem. Sources of worry to him are his being off work, financial problems, and crowded conditions at home. He worries that he may be permanently disabled. He always considered himself a robust, healthy man but has seen himself change physically over the past few years and can no longer do some of the things he had been able to before. Source of income—unemployment. Health insurance—partial coverage of inpatient care by private company.

Such a profile does not lengthen a patient's chart unduly. It gives clinicians a respectful, yet revealing description of the human being they are treating. Above all, it avoids the degrading travesty of a "social history" that one so often sees scrawled in a patient's chart—"Smokes two ppd. Etoh mod."

TAKING NOTES

The issue of whether to take notes at the bedside, and how extensively, has implications for patient care. Students will find educators who make recommendations at both extremes. The advantages of taking notes at the bedside are obvious. No one has a perfect memory, and a good, accurate depiction of dates, events, and chronology is critical to a good medical history. The hazards, however, are twofold. First, a physician who is constantly looking at his notepad is not looking at his patient. It is amazing to watch the number of things that doctors manage to hold up in front of themselves to avoid patient contact. We have seen physicians who cannot even enter the room with a patient unless "armed" with a chart, several exotic instruments, and a handy i.v. pole. Burying oneself in notes can be a similar distancing device. Second, there is something to be said for a degree of passive receptiveness when listening to a patient. If one does not try so hard to concentrate on details, one often learns a great deal that is important. One is far more apt to be tuned into the moods, subtle mannerisms, nuances, and even smells that give clues to the patient's problem. The more that one is trying to structure and record as one goes along, the less apt one is to pick up on the patient's gestalt. Despite this, we recommend that the student take some notes at the bedside. Accuracy *is* very important, and many clinicians can lull themselves into thinking that their memory will be better 24 hours later than in fact it is. Especially when obtaining the chronology of illness, we suggest that the student jot down pertinent notes, restricting them to the essential dates, names, and salient facts that he will need to enhance his recall later. In other words, notes should be as parsimonious as possible, the minimum needed to help one recall and record the medical history more thoroughly at a later time, preferably within 12 hours, because letting the matter go much longer defeats the purpose of brief, orienting notes.

RECORDING THE MEDICAL HISTORY

Developing an ability to record the medical history in concise, grammatically correct, legible English is a basic medical skill. It is also one that is abysmally substandard in many clinicians.

An essential part of our interviewing course at the University of Colorado is the student's medical write-up. Each student is expected to prepare a number of histories for his preceptor's evaluation and critique. Critique can focus on issues of content—excessive length, errors, excessive brevity—but also commonly includes mundane issues of grammar, gross misspelling, and dangling participles. The goal is not to harass students about punctuation and grammar. On the other hand, accurate, intelligible recording of data is a critical skill that requires practice and one that should be formed early in the student's education.

PRESENTING THE HISTORY

During the 3rd and 4th years of medical school and continuing into postgraduate training, a great deal of clinical teaching will be done on "rounds." "Rounds" is a medical colloquialism for any gathering of doctors during which communications about patients are verbally shared. These can range from informal bedside-to-bedside checks, conducted with a senior house officer, to more elaborate, ritualized affairs. These latter events are often referred to as "presenting to the attending." Typically, a more experienced clinician, often a senior faculty member, will hear a student present a patient's case in depth. This is done in front of other students, interns, residents, and members of the treatment team and is traditionally followed by an examination of the patient at the bedside. This teaching technique, originally popularized by Sir William Osler, has survived as a major form of medical communication and education to the present. There is nothing more disheartening than the sight of 10 or 20 clinicians suddenly crowding into a patient's room, brushing aside relatives, and "presenting" a patient in a way that is dehumanizing, filled with jargon, and often terrifying to the patient. Similarly, some attendings seem to feel that students and house officers are best taught by techniques of humiliation and stress. These are what students often refer to as "why didn't you?" rounds: the hapless student, intern, or resident is roasted over the coals by his attending about sins of omission and commission, articles not read, and lab values not instantly accessible. What this kind of ritual has to do with good patient care, much less medical education or even common courtesy, is not clear. In fact, how a student or resident treated in such an insensitive way can be expected to in turn consistently relate to his patients with compassion is beyond the wisdom of these authors.

Leaving aside these abuses, which are common enough that the student should be warned about them, presenting patients verbally is a critical skill. It is essential to be able to communicate succinctly and accurately to colleagues about a given patient. Therefore, we encourage students in our interviewing course to refine this ability early by practicing at presenting their cases. This is surprisingly stressful, even in a small group that has developed rapport over time. Most of us have a bit of "stage fright" when it comes to presenting. Needless to say, we advocate that the student be permitted to practice this important skill in an atmosphere of support and encouragement. It is our experience that rudeness and degradation teach little, unless one's goals are to educate clinicians in the defenses of callousness and nihilism.

During this chapter we have described the basic components of the medical history and the place that this information assumes in the overall recording of data in a patient's chart. We have elaborated the particular importance of the history of present illness and touched briefly on the importance of beginning to develop skills in recording and presenting patients' medical histories verbally. In Chapter 9, we will shift from the final product—the components themselves—to the process of obtaining that product. It is here that the art and science of medicine truly converge.

References

Hiller, A. (Dir.): *Hospital*, script by Paddy Chayefsky, United Artists, 1971.

Morgan, W.L., and Engel, G.L.: *The Clinical Approach to the Patient*, W.B. Sanders Co. Philadelphia, 1969.

Platt, F.W., and McMath, J.C.: Clinical hypocompetence: The interview. *Ann. Intern. Med. 91:* 898, 1979.

Schwartz, M.: Personal communication.

chapter 9

OBTAINING THE MEDICAL HISTORY

OBTAINING A HISTORY IS A COLLABORATION

As is true of the entire patient-physician relationship, the process of obtaining a medical history requires a collaboration between doctor and patient. The physician, no matter how skilled, cannot simply extract a history from his patient. The patient, no matter how articulate, cannot give a history in final form without help and guidance from the physician. The process of obtaining a history can be fruitfully compared to the relationship that exists in modern space flight between ground control and a crew of astronauts aboard a rocket ship.

Imagine the physician as "ground control," equipped with all the most sophisticated tracking devices (interviewing skills) and computerized guidance systems (clinical experience and knowledge of pathophysiology). In turn, imagine the patient as a crew of astronauts aboard a rocket, sending signals (the history as the patient perceives it) and awaiting guidance (the physician's ability to distill these communications and direct his patient's further communications accordingly). In such a collaboration, ground control and astronauts together would guide the rocket toward its objective (obtaining a history).

In this example, each set of data sent to earth would constantly be refined; the process of input and analysis would continuously yield more and more specific information, prompting ever more precise alterations in the rocket's course (sharpening the details of the history). While detailed inspection of the ship's course would show many momentary alterations, the overall final course would appear smooth and consistent. The physician is a sophisticated guidance system, equipped with a heart. Combining technical knowledge with compassion and human understanding, he obtains the medical history through skillful facilitating, attentive listening, and empathic silence.

Up to this point in the book, we have examined the foundation of all interviewing: the milieu of feelings in which both interviewer and patient participate and the mutual process of communicating. We will now examine the bridge between process and content—how the verbal and nonverbal process communications between doctor and patient can be refined into a medical history. We will stress the rationale for approaching the history from the standpoint of formulating problems, emphasizing how such problems can be defined and developed within the traditional format of the medical history already presented in Chapter 8.

INTERVIEWING AND THE PROBLEM ORIENTED MEDICAL RECORD

Students in our curriculum at the University of Colorado do their first few interviews in a supportive atmosphere where they are asked to deal mainly with process issues, i.e., how the illness is affecting the life of a patient, what the emotional tone of an interview is, and how the student and patient respond to each other. As students become familiar with this kind of interviewing, they quickly progress to a more content-oriented phase of the course and concentrate on techniques of eliciting medical information and developing an account of the present illness. There is also opportunity in this phase to practice write-ups and verbal presentations. Not surprisingly, students experience some discomfort and anxiety during this transition. Here, it can be helpful for them to realize that they are learning in a very special and fertile environment: they have the luxury of interviewing, free from the weighty responsibility for therapeutic decisions. This relationship to patients is unique to students in interviewing courses and can be used to their advantage.

Students also find this transition easier when they can conceptualize the place of the medical history in the overall management of patients. Where, then, does the history fit, and how can it be obtained in a professional and caring manner? The answer, we believe, lies in great part in an understanding of the Problem Oriented Medical Record (POMR) as developed by Lawrence Weed.

In his clinical work, Dr. Weed was struck by the confusion he discerned in traditional medical records, which he found to be unscientific, haphazard, and unauditable. He therefore developed a new system for recording medical data called the Problem Oriented Medical Record. The POMR is a comprehensive approach to all aspects of clinical thinking and patient care—not simply a record-keeping system. Students being educated today can expect to hear a great deal about this system during their training, and we will not attempt to cover the subject definitively here. We do wish to introduce the subject at this point, however, because the POMR is fundamentally a conceptual tool; it provides a sense of direction in the history-taking process not only for the beginning student but also for the experienced practitioner.

The Four Phases of Medical Action

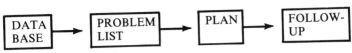

In the POMR, Weed conceptualized all of medical action as having four connected and interdependent phases. These phases represent the thought processes through which diagnosis is reached and treatment plans are formulated. This diagnostic process is an integral part of the interview process itself. In Chapter 6, we discussed how the interaction between patient and doctor shapes the flow and sequence of the interview. Here, the clinician's thinking shapes the flow and sequence of the medical history in a similar manner.

Phase I—The Data Base

The data base is composed of the *medical history*, the *physical examination*, and *laboratory information*. It includes all information in these areas discovered about the patient from the first time he presented himself for medical care to the present.

The data base has several qualities. It is *generative*: the more information asked for, the more extensive the physical examination, the better the history, the *more data* that will be obtained. It is *creative*: a seemingly infinite number of questions, physical examination maneuvers, and laboratory tests could be performed; yet it is through creative integration and synthesis of all available and potential data that the data base develops into its best form. It is *variable*: the data base is variable depending on the specialty of the physician. For example, an opthalmologist might ask as many as 30 questions in reviewing the visual system, while an internist would ask only 3 or 4. It is variable from clinician to clinician, even in the same specialty. A skilled clinician can obtain a vastly different data base from the same patient than can someone less skilled. Finally, the data base is variable over time. The *same* clinician can obtain a very different data base from the *same* patient on two different occasions. In spite of many attempts to define a standardized data base (often age and gender specific), no such standard exists. Often, health care institutions define standardized data bases (such as multiphasic screening), but these are trial-and-error approaches based loosely on poorly justifiable medical and cost-effectiveness considerations. Every clinician must accept and contend with this inexactitude in the data base. It is possible, however, to define standard minimum requirements, as we did for the medical history in Chapter 8 and in the Appendix.

Phase II—The Problem List

From the data base gathered in history taking, a clinician must formulate a list of his patient's specific problems. In doing so, it is especially important

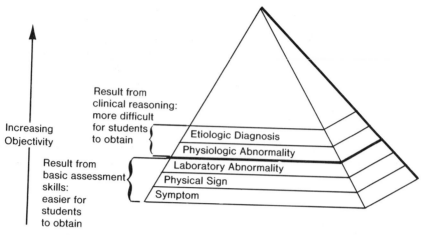

Diagram 9.1   Illustration adapted from A.E. Voytovich.

to know how to rank the problems on a scale of increasing objectivity. The pyramid in Diagram 9.1 proposes such a schema by identifying problems according to five basic categories, arranged in increasing levels of objectivity: a *symptom*, a *physical sign*, a *laboratory abnormality* (such as hyperglycemia or T wave inversion V_{4-6} on the electrocardiogram), a *physiologic abnormality* (such as congestive heart failure, hypertension, or asthma), and a specific *etiologic diagnosis* (such as congestive heart failure due to rheumatic heart disease or oat cell carcinoma of the left lower lobe of the lung). Many clinicians add a sixth category of problem, *psychosocial abnormality*, which includes such problems as "battered wife" or "chronic anxiety over functional problems." This sixth category clearly does not fit neatly into the pyramid yet is essential and must be included in a good work-up. The problem list thus defines all non-trivial abnormalities disclosed by a thorough search of the data base.

One great advantage of the problem list for the student lies in its adaptability to a broad range of clinical knowledge and experience. Under older systems of record keeping, the physician was expected to record his "impression" i.e., his best guess as to the etiology of the patient's presenting problem. This can be very difficult for a student, who may be able to recognize symptoms and laboratory values that are abnormal, for instance, but not necessarily know what diagnosis they represent. By contrast, the POMR is adaptable to each clinician's level of certainty, as illustrated in the following example.

A student, having worked up his patient, presented the following problem list to his preceptor:

Problems

1. Dyspnea on exertion   (a symptom)
2. Nocturia   (a symptom)
3. Pedal edema   (a sign)

4. S_3 gallop   (a sign)
5. Cardiomegaly by chest x-ray   (a lab abnormality)

The student had been quite complete and accurate in his data collection—there were no other abnormalities to be found in the data base by review or rechecking the patient. He was also clearly defining his level of understanding, and it was then easy for his preceptor to condense the patient's problem list into a single physiologic diagnosis:

Congestive heart failure

When several problems can be condensed with confidence into a single problem of greater objective certainty, this should be done. In this example, the student's preceptor was able to do so instantly. When several problems cannot be condensed in this way (either because of the student's limited experience or the complexity of the problem), the POMR permits the clinician to record his impressions at his own level of understanding. The educational advantage of this can be substantial. In this example, the preceptor was able to immediately identify the cutting edge of this student's knowledge and understanding and thereby know how to teach at an appropriate level. The inherent auditability of such a problem list is also clear.

Phase III—The Plan

The systematic attack for each problem is spelled out in the plan. There is a plan *for each problem*, and it consists of three parts: a *diagnostic plan*, a *therapeutic plan*, and a *patient education plan*. It is a clear statement of what we will do for *this* problem in *this* person at *this* time. Accountability and auditability are glorified in the plan. It is appropriate, for example, as part of the diagnostic plan to see, "Read more about this disease" or "Don't understand this clearly—will seek consultation." No one expects total recall or encyclopedic knowledge from students; rather, one hopes to give them the tools to solve problems and to attempt logical approaches. The patient education portion of the plan is an area in which the clinician spells out the patient's understanding of the problem and the treatment plan and suggests areas in which the patient needs more education. It is especially useful for a patient with a fatal or severely disabling illness to record that patient's understanding and acceptance of the treatment process.

It is sometimes difficult for beginning students to think seriously about diagnostic and therapeutic plans for the patients they interview. The stakes are simply not so high as they will be later on, when clinical responsibilities are increased. Yet, from the outset, students can appreciate how ongoing considerations of a plan will be very much on a clinician's mind as he is gathering data in the medical history. Most students, in fact, have the thought at times during introductory interviews, "Someday a patient like this will be mine; someday my responsibilities for him will be very real."

Phase IV—The Follow-Up

Follow-up refers back to the original problems: it begs the questions, "do we do what we say we will do?" When clinicians record their thinking regarding follow-up in the medical record, they do so in a four-part entry for each problem: *subjective* (new historical data), *objective* (laboratory and physical examination data), *assessment* (a brief, coherent formulation of the problem and its most likely etiologies), and *plan* (in three parts to show what further diagnostic, treatment, and educational plans are to be accomplished). This format is usually referred to by the mnemonic "SOAP," referring to the follow-up's four components of subjective data, objective data, assessment, and plan. Reviewing a sequence of progress notes recorded in this fashion will often reveal forgotten tests, unfulfilled therapeutic trials, and inadequate teaching. This is unfortunate, but human. The advantage to this system is that it makes such errors readily discernible and, therefore, amenable to correction.

Students up on the wards early in their training are naturally not going to feel the sense of immediacy regarding follow-up that they will feel later. As was true for the *plan*, considerations of follow-up initially seem quite remote. This sense of detachment, which leads some students to complain that interviewing courses are contrived and artificial, can be reduced by providing students with opportunities to follow the patients they interview under supervision. This lends a much greater air of reality to interviewing, and most students say that it enhances their sense of professional purpose. When such experiences are not possible, it is still valuable to encourage students to think about what they would do to follow up a problem. Actual entries in the patient's chart may still be a year or two away, but students can be helped to anticipate these responsibilities from the outset.

In summary, we believe that an overview of the POMR is useful for students from the outset. Though they will not initially be applying it directly to the patient's written medical record, it is valuable as a conceptual tool—anchoring interviewing skills more meaningfully in the overall objectives of medical care. We can obviously not do full justice to the POMR in an introduction such as the one presented here, so we refer the reader to an excellent book by Hurst and Walker (see references) that fully defines the POMR and explores its uses and ramifications.

THE ELEMENTS COMMON TO ALL HISTORIES (SOTN)

In Part II of this book we discussed at some length how a patient can be encouraged to open up and communicate more about himself, primarily through techniques that evolve naturally from an understanding of the interview *process*. In Chapter 8, we described Morgan and Engel's seven dimensions of illness—an eminently useful schema for organizing and describing a variety of symptoms. Most students find that when they are armed with an understanding of process and a grasp of the seven dimensions, they can begin to organize their thinking about the medical history. Yet, these two tools alone, as valuable as they are, still seem insufficient at times when students attempt to sort out the masses of content data that patients report during the medical history. The seven dimensions do not fit all symptoms equally well. Moreover, many of the patients that students see in university hospitals and tertiary care settings have complex prior medical histories. Students understandably feel a need for a system of thinking and organization applicable to these more complicated patients.

To this end, we propose another way to organize historical information, a framework that is conceptually somewhat broader than the seven dimensions and intended to complement them. This organizational framework is abbreviated SOTN and stands for the four elements common to all medical problems: *subjective* data, *objective* data, *therapeutic* data, and *significant negatives.*

Subjective Data

Subjective data include all information conveyed directly by the patient. The clinician may often choose to translate it into medical terms but the information itself comes from the patient. As such, it is inherently judgmental in nature, emotionally laden, and slanted by the patient's anxieties, perceptions, and priorities. This information *depends upon* the patient's interpretation and recall of events. It ranges from simple description to a complex history, from 2 days of vomiting in a previously healthy college student to a decade-long history of renal failure in an elderly woman, with consequent symptoms in almost every organ system, numerous medical complications, and countless treatment side effects. Subjective information is always filtered through the prism of a patient's own unique fears and wishes. Usually, this is obvious, and it is no less true of the highly educated patient. Consider the physician as patient, for example. While he would probably give information that is more technical and clinically focused, it would still be highly subjective; the physician as *patient* is just as frightened and prone to denial as anyone else. He may use his technical knowledge to mask his feelings of vulnerability from himself, but his doctor must not fall into the same trap.

Except for the occasional physician patient, most people naturally express themselves in non-technical language. It is therefore the clinician's task to cull the essential meaning of his patient's account of illness and distill it into concise, accurate medical terminology. This is a skill that develops during medical school but that is refined during the years of house staff training. For example, "shortness of breath that the patient says he first noticed about a year ago when he climbed a flight of stairs, which has now gotten much worse so that he doesn't even have to move around to get winded," may be restated: "A 1-year history of light dyspnea on exertion which has progressed to dyspnea at rest." The essence of the information has thus been condensed but still captured.

There is a huge professional vocabulary to be mastered, and it is important for the student to be exposed to it early in his training. During medical school, the student will learn literally thousands of words, such as pleuritic, hematemesis, bitemporal, epigastric, dyspareunia, and dyspnea. Mastering a thorough medical vocabulary helps physicians to record subjective information concisely and to communicate it in a commonly understood language to other professionals.

Objective Data

Objective information in the history is composed of documented physical signs, laboratory results, or other measureable information. It is relatively "hard data," subject to interpretation regarding its meaning but not its presence. An enlarged liver, an elevated blood sugar, and the results of an x-ray are examples of objective information. The weight, blood pressure, or amount of edema are other examples. This type of information may be recounted by the patient himself—"The doctor said my coronary arteriography showed a block in the main vessel of the heart"—but is considered definitely objective only when verified by chart review, e.g., "80% narrowing of the left main coronary artery proximally." In fact, most objective data are (or should be) available from the medical record. They can often best be presented in flow sheet form, quite appropriate for a present illness for which past history includes many tests over a long period.

Therapeutic Data

The treatment of the problem—by the medical community, the patient himself, or others—is always relevant to the history of any problem. Treatment may range from specific medications (including dosages, length of treatment, side effects, and adverse reactions) to surgical procedures or to the incantations and ministrations of a faith healer. It is all relevant and frequently yields diagnostic information, as in the case of Dr. Reiser's "colitis" described in Chapter 3.

We must also remember that the history of how a patient has previously tried to get treatment tells us a great deal, in process, about that person, and describes the milestones in the chronology of the illness, the patient's perception of the seriousness and cause of the illness, and the progression and regression of symptoms over time (e.g., due to medication or placebo, whose powerful effects must always be considered). This type of clinical thinking, which becomes *part of the interviewing process* itself, is often called "differential diagnosis" or "clinical reasoning." Sound clinical thinking certainly includes these skills, yet it is not summed up by them. The fact that computers can be programmed to do this type of "thinking" proves that logic is involved. But, the logic of a truly skilled clinician is not so easily reduced to programmable effects; an intangible synergism of logic, intuition, common sense, and empathy operates in a skilled clinician's mind in a way that cannot be duplicated by a computer; and it is in the clinical interview, based on a good doctor-patient relationship, that clinical reasoning develops to fullest fruition.

Significant Negatives

What does not occur in the course of an illness can be as important as what does. This type of information—the pertinent negatives—helps a clinician to determine *how* sick a patient is as well as in what way. Often, a most difficult yet critical clinical task involves deciding when a person is well. It is easy to recognize the very sick and the very healthy; but between these two extremes lie the early sick and the worried well. Negatives help us evaluate these patients by answering the questions: "What is the most serious condition that will explain these symptoms in this person?" and "What common or uncommon condition(s) present like this?"

When a patient complains of chest pain, for example, significant negatives include the fact that the pain is *not* brought on by exercise or relieved by rest, is *not* squeezing or crushing, and does *not* radiate to the jaws or left arm. In general, significant negatives are all the important symptoms of a given organ system that a patient denies. Sometimes a review of negatives requires that the clinician cover more than one organ system, as in the case of certain multisystem diseases, such as diabetes and autoimmune syndromes. Generally, knowing what can go seriously wrong in each organ system enables a clinician to know what is important in a history by its *absence*. This clinical ability is closely linked to a clinician's level of experience and knowledge of pathophysiology. The Review of Systems, described in the Appendix, can serve as a guide to pertinent negatives in a given organ system. As we pointed out in Chapter 8, in fact, if one has taken a thorough history, including negatives, most of the review of systems obtained at the end of the interview should not divulge any new pertinent data.

A word of caution: do not obtain a history of significant negatives by asking questions *in the negative*. For instance, never put words into the patient's mouth by asking, "The pain wasn't squeezing in nature, was it?" This type of question implies an expected response in the negative and will often be answered that way simply to please the interviewer. Negatively phrased questions may also inadvertently instill considerable fear in a patient, who will wonder if a positive response implies something dire: "I wonder why the Doctor asked that? It must be because I have ————!" (Fill in the blank with a serious or fatal illness of the patient's choosing.) It is usually best to begin a line of inquiry with open-ended questions, gradually tapering down to questions that ask for key negatives in a more specific, directed way. The student should also be cautioned about the danger of reading lists of symptoms to a patient because they may distract and confuse the patient with an array of "multiple choice" questions.

In the example that follows, a patient has complained of shortness of breath. The student wonders if chest pain might also be present and obtains the history in a way that very effectively establishes the presence of pertinent negatives.

Student: Do you have any other symptoms while you are short of breath?

Patient: Yes, I sweat.
   S: Any other feelings?
   P: No.
   S: Have you ever noticed dizziness?
   P: No.
   S: Palpitations?
   P: No.
   S: Chest pain?
   P: No.

The student could have said, "Have you ever noted dizziness, palpitations, or chest pain?" (a list), but this would be far less acceptable. Here, he has pinned down three very significant negatives in this patient's history. Had the patient responded positively to his question about chest pain, he might have gone on to establish the *quality* of that pain and its other dimensions. Thus,

   S: Can you tell me more about the chest pain?
   P: It hurts a lot!
   S: What does it feel like?
   P: It just hurts, it's hard to say.
   S: If you had to choose whether the pain felt more like burning, aching, stabbing, or pressure which would you choose?
   P: Aching.
   S: Aching?
   P: Yes, like a toothache.
   S: Is it ever a pressure feeling?
   P: No.

In the first case, the student would write, "The patient denies dizziness, palpitations, and chest pain." In the second case, "The patient complains of an aching chest pain, but denies a squeezing, burning, or stabbing quality."

A clinician will sometimes search out different significant negatives, depending on the age, sex, and clinical status of the patient. For instance, significant negatives for a young woman with chest pain who is taking birth control pills include denial of pleuritic type pain. In a 51-year-old business executive with chest pain, angina pectoris may be strongly suspected, and pertinent negatives would include the denial of a squeezing, pressure-like quality to the pain. To reiterate, a history of negatives is important to rule in or rule out specific serious illnesses. If pulmonary embolism is suspected in a young female patient, a negative history of pleuritic chest pain will be crucial. In an older male business executive, the same chief complaint, chest pain, will lead the clinician to search for symptoms associated with angina (i.e., pain from myocardial ischemia).

Here is an example of a write-up based on the SOTN approach. We have identified its components on the left:

Subjective   The patient was in his usual state of health until 3 days ago
                      when he developed persistent vomiting of all oral intake except
                      for sips of water. He vomited approximately four times a day

	and noted epigastric burning pain and lower abdominal cramping pain just prior to vomiting.
Objective	Two days ago the patient was seen in clinic where a white count and physical exam were normal.
Therapeutic	He was given a clear liquid diet and Compazine 5 mg q. 6 h. without relief.
Subjective	All symptoms persisted to the present with the addition, for the past 24 hours, of six episodes of mucus containing diarrhea and fever to 103°.
Negatives	The patient denies hematemesis, melena, hematochezia, rigor, travel outside the U.S., close exposure to others with similar symptoms, weight loss, constipation, or similar symptoms in the past.

This report of a patient's current problem is a good example of the appropriate use of the SOTN framework to develop a concise and accurate account of viral gastroenteritis. Moreover, the report demonstrates another important tool—the clinician's ability to organize the four kinds of data in chronological order. The use of chronology as a key organizer was discussed in Chapter 8 and will be elaborated later in this chapter under Practical Approaches to the Patient.

THE "A.R.T." OF INTERVIEWING—A BRIDGE BETWEEN CONTENT AND PROCESS

How does a clinician get the vital information he needs without disrupting the natural flow of a patient's spontaneous associations during the interview—a spontaneity so essential to an understanding of that person and to the building of rapport? Put another way, how can a clinician learn to "follow" his patient, staying with him empathically, without being hopelessly diverted into an excursion where the patient decides what to bring up (and not bring up) and the clinician loses all sense of direction and control? Most students find that they conduct interviews at both extremes—being "led by the nose" in one interview, only to be too controlling in the next.

Striking a balance is difficult. In fact, we regard this balance, which involves building an effective bridge between interviewing's process and content, as one of the most difficult skills a clinician has to master.

What follows in this section is a proposal regarding the steps by which we believe such a balance is struck when the clinician is effective. What we describe here is not offered as a conscious strategy to be applied cookbook fashion by the interviewer. In fact, clinicians who consistently strike this balance apply these steps quite unconsciously. We believe there is value in objectifying them, however, since most clinicians (and students) find this bridge between content and process so difficult to effect with grace.

Just as all human interactions have a process, they can also be viewed as having three overlapping and highly reciprocal phases: *Assessment, Ranking,* and *Transition.* Each of these can occur at a verbal or nonverbal level and may be within a person's awareness or unconscious. To give a simple example: A door-to-door salesman wishes to sell a set of encyclopedias to a housewife. As soon as she opens the door, each begins to assess the other. The salesman is thinking, does she look receptive or is she going to be a hardnose? He may be peering over her shoulder to size up the furniture in the foyer—does the family seem to have the money it takes to buy a set of encyclopedias? Similarly, the housewife is sizing up the salesman—is he ethical? Is he offering a good product, or is he just a con-artist? Their words to each other will contribute to their mutual assessment; but, a great deal will go on at the intuitive, "hunch," level. Each of them will begin to *rank* his or her assessments almost immediately. The salesman may, for example, decide that he'd better deal with the scowl on his perspective client's face and her tendency to shut the door before he describes the wonders of his encyclopedia. "Is that your little boy playing in the living room?" he may begin. "How cute. He looks like a bright little fellow!" The housewife, in turn, will be ranking her preceptions as well. Does he look trustworthy enough to even be let in the door? Should she give him a chance with his "spiel," but listen with skepticism? Finally, the interaction will progress through *transitions.* The salesman may say, "Before I tell you more, might I come in and show you just *one* of these lovely full color brochures?" The housewife may already be signalling transitions through body language (closing the door, scowling) or direct expression, for instance, looking at her watch and saying, "I'm sorry but I really must be going, I have another appointment."

There is a useful analogy between this example and the doctor-patient relationship. In both, the three phases of the interaction occur quickly and simultaneously. A great deal of rapport building or rapport destruction will occur very early, long before either party achieves a level of collaboration that will permit them to "get down to business." As any successful encyclopedia salesman knows, in fact, two-thirds of the battle will be won with a customer before he even gets the samples out of the valise. Similarly, in the doctor-patient relationship, a great deal of important assessment, ranking, and transition will take place before getting into the heart of the medical history.

The analogy is not perfect—in most cases, the doctor does not have to persuade his patient to let him offer his product (though occasionally this will occur). Furthermore, most patients place an inherently high level of trust in the doctor-patient interaction that will accelerate the speed at which both can get down to the content-directed medical history. Finally, the vulnerability and anxiety of illness itself brings on a uniquely altered state of consciousness in which patients are especially prone to freely discuss their personal matters with a physician. Despite these differences, however, the similarities should be obvious. A physician is going to have to sell himself, at the process level, if he is to obtain a reliable history, developed in an atmosphere of trust that will also permit future meaningful collaboration.

Although "A.R.T." is acutally a *mutual* process, in the following discussion we will describe it from the doctor's perspective, with particular attention to aspects of interviewing, decision-making, and technique that result from this perspective.

Assessment

Assessment is the phase of the interview in which the clinician is maximally open-minded, receptive, and non-directive. Its goal is to elicit as many associations about as many concerns in the patient as possible. In practice, this phase may last only seconds to minutes; yet, it is a critical phase of the data gathering process. From here, the clinician quickly moves into *ranking*, but throughout the interview assessment continues as an active process, and the clinician always tries to listen with a third ear.

The key to accuracy during the assessment phase of the medical interview lies in one's ability to maintain a relaxed receptiveness. The stance is far less active than a student might initially expect: a seasoned clinician will have his eyes open and his senses alert, but he will be relatively quiet. Especially during the initial phase of his interview, he will allow his mind to wander. He might find himself noticing an odor; he may be struck by the unusual color of a patient's hair; he may be curious about a certain expression that he notices on his patient's face. As the patient's story begins to unfold, many thoughts will cross the physician's mind—memories of other patients, random associations to journal articles, diseases, and syndromes. As the interview progresses and becomes more focused, the clinician's attention will progressively become more active and directed. The bits and pieces of data he has been gathering from the patient begin to converge toward a diagnostic hypothesis, and he will be focusing his attention with increasing intensity. The process is somewhat analogous to that of a bird hunter in the field. Long before the bird (the diagnosis) is spotted by the hunter (the doctor), the hunter will amble along, allowing his eyes to roam freely across the horizon, taking in the sights and enjoying the breezes, smells, and sounds. It will be in this state of relaxed receptiveness that he is most apt to spot a bird. Were he craning his neck at every bush and peering into every tree, he would be far less likely to achieve success. Then, something will catch his attention. He may hear a rustling or just sense something. He will begin to hunt down the bird more deliberately now (akin to a later stage of the medical interview when the physician is focusing in on the diagnosis). By the end of the process, when the hunter has actually spotted his bird, his attention will be riveted on a very precise location, as will the physician's at an analogous point. However, even at a very advanced stage of the clinical interview, a skilled physician will keep at least one part of his mind hovering freely—relaxed and receptive—ready to be taken by surprise; assessment is a continuous process.

To put a patient at ease and so ensure his openness to expressing any and all of his concerns during the assessment phase of the interview, the clinician should begin the discussion in a general, non-directed way. For years, psychiatrists have known the importance of beginning with a non-leading question. This is just as advisable for the medical interview. The student should begin his interview with a question such as, "What sort of troubles have you been having?" Or a simple nod and an encouraging gesture of the hand may tell the patient that the clinician is ready to listen to whatever the patient wishes to say. The purpose of such openings is not to play "stone-faced psychiatrist," but rather to permit the patient to start with *his* concerns, whatever they are. For instance, even the seemingly bland and innocuous opening used by many physicians—"What brings you to the hospital?"— implies that the patient *should* focus his concerns on the present illness. Certainly this will be important, but a physician should never communicate to a patient that he is interested only in the patient's disease.

Here is a brief clinical vignette that illustrates the process of assessment. You will notice that the physician begins the encounter with an entirely open-ended question.

> Mrs. Anderson is a 59-year-old woman admitted to the hospital because of fever, chills, and pain in the right upper quadrant of her abdomen. When the clinician first walks in the room, he notices that she is staring rather wistfully out the window. She holds a damp kleenex in her right hand. Upon hearing the doctor's knock at her open door, she immediately turns, puts on a cheery smile, and says "Come on in! Come on in!" Her next remark, before the clinician has had a chance to introduce himself, is "My you look so young! You doctors seem so young nowadays!"
>
> After introducing himself appropriately, the doctor asks, "What sort of troubles have you been having?"
>
> P: Oh, nothing serious, I suppose. The doctor thinks it's just trouble with my gallbladder. (Patient sighs.)
> D: Your gall bladder?
> P: Yes, he thinks that's what it is. They're in here to take the bag out of the old baggage—that's the way I put it anyway. (Patient lets forth with a hollow chuckle.)

From this open-ended beginning, the clinician has been able to assess several concerns immediately: the possibility of gall bladder disease, an underlying mood of sadness that the patient tries to hide through hollow humor, concerns about the doctor's age, the possibility of upcoming surgery, and lowered self-esteem ("take the bag out of the old baggage"). Had the physician not been able to maintain a stance of relaxed receptiveness at the outset, he might have missed her tears, which she quickly tried to hide. Similarly, it is easy to see how, with too medically-focused an opening, this patient would obligingly launch into a detailed history of her gall bladder symptoms, without alluding to her other concerns.

Ranking

Once the initial assessment has begun, the clinician immediately begins to rank his priorities. Again, this can be a largely unconscious process, yet it goes on constantly. Ranking is based on clinical experience, medical urgency, and a clinician's style. Too many clinicians rank rigidly, almost automatically subordinating everything to the medical problem—an approach that we feel is ill-advised.

In some situations, of course, the medical problem must be ranked first. If a 60-year-old man is brought to the emergency room by ambulance complaining of severe chest pain and an irregular beating of his heart, the physician must begin with a rapid history of present illness, focusing on coronary symptoms. Such a patient may well be concerned about many things: getting to work the next day, calling his children to tell them he has arrived, or wanting to know how much the hospital will cost. Despite these concerns that the patient may express quite insistently, the physician obviously ranks the medical emergency as preeminent.

In most situations, however, there is less urgency, and the clinician has far more latitude in ranking his interview priorities. This is how the clinician, cited in the previous example of the lady with gallbladder disease, ranked his own priorities with this patient. He did not do this consciously, incidentally, but he was able to reconstruct his reasoning when specifically asked. He decided that depression and low self-esteem seemed to be a pervading concern. "The sadness in the room was so thick, you could cut it," he said. Yet, he said that he "sensed" that if "I came on too strong about depression, that might turn her off, too." Therefore he decided to rank his priorities in the following sequence. (1) Begin by establishing better alliance; find out more about the patient, her life, who she is. (2) This will probably lead into the depression. She should have a chance to talk about this before being directed too specifically to the medical problem. (3) Then explore the possibility of gall bladder disease or other illness. (4) Concerns about my age; my hunch is this will take care of itself if rapport is established.

One can see that a great deal of clinical intuition and experience go into this kind of ranking. In fact, a large number of intuitive expressions are used by the clinician to describe how he ranked his priorities—he *felt* a depression in the room, he had a *hunch* that he shouldn't approach it too directly. Despite the complexity and subtlety of this process, however, it has been our experience that most students have the natural aptitude to rank in this manner; the task is to teach them how to trust their own intuitive processes.

Transitions

The clinician's ability to effect smooth transitions in the interview is of great importance. Patients generally tolerate a wide variety of interviewing styles and accommodate themselves to many different kinds of clinicians. The clinician's ability to effect smooth transitions, however, can make the difference between a bewildering, choppy experience for the patient and one in which empathy and collaboration flow between doctor and patient.

Effecting transitions is fairly simple, if one remembers to do it. It requires no special oratorical grace but does require the clinician's willingness to inform his patient of when and why transitions in the interview are occurring.

Not only is this one of the easier techniques of medical interviewing, it is also one of the most frequently overlooked. It is essential to remember that the patient cannot read your mind and, as a non-physician, will usually not be able to follow the train of your thought. Therefore, make sure that you *share* your thinking aloud with the patient.

Here is how it worked in the clinical example we have been discussing:

P: They're in here to take the bag out of the old baggage . . . "
D: Hmm, I see . . . You know, I'm going to want to hear more about this gall bladder problem, and especially get the information from you firsthand. But before we get into that, could you tell me a little bit more about yourself. (Pause) Are you from this area?
P: (With a sigh) No. I only recently moved out here, from Minneapolis. I'm staying with my oldest daughter and her husband.

From here, the patient was able to go on to express a number of very painful concerns. Her husband had died the previous year. The patient, feeling depressed, lonely, and helpless, had essentially been on the road ever since, staying with different children and relatives. This made her feel dependent and like a free loader; yet she felt too lonely and afraid of her grief to return to the house in which she lived with her husband. The interviewer's ability to elicit this material was based on his ability to assess its presence, to rank it as a matter of importance, and then to communicate to his patient through transition what he was asking, when, and why. Later in the interview, after the patient had shared a great deal with him, he felt the need to return to the problem of his patient's gallbladder.

P: . . . so that's quite a story anyway, huh?
D: It certainly is! It sounds like it's been a pretty painful year. I *am* going to shift gears at this point a bit, however, and return to the business of your gallbladder. Can you tell me more about the symptoms you've been having.
P: Well mostly it's been fever, some chills, and this pain. . . .

We have described these three phases of the interview process in a linear fashion—showing how one leads into the next. In fact, the process is not exactly linear, it is more like an ascending spiral of ever decreasing diameter. In other words, assessment and ranking usually lead to further assessment and ranking. Throughout the process, the clinician performs these mental operations rapidly and without much conscious awareness. This may be one reason why clinicians so frequently neglect to inform their patients of shifts, by providing adequate transitions. Effecting transitions is the most *conscious* part of the process and is based on a simple principle: share what you're thinking with the patient. To return, finally, to an earlier example—the businessman brought to the emergency room with chest pain and an irregular heart beat—the clinician here clearly does not have time to develop a leisurely social history/patient profile. He does have the time, however, to share with his patient the reason for not doing so in the form of a transition: "It sounds like there're going to be a lot of loose ends we'll have to help you take care of tonight, Mr. Jones, but I *do* want to start with your chest pain, since that sounds like it's been pretty bad for the last couple of hours and maybe we ought to start there."

PRACTICAL APPROACHES TO THE PATIENT

In this section, we will consider three situations that students commonly encounter when they interview patients and offer suggestions for how they can be handled most effectively.

Guiding Chronology

As we have stressed, chronology is a key parameter in developing meaningful historical information. Yet, most patients do not view chronology from the same perspective that we do as clinicians. To illustrate this, pause for a moment and recall the past year's events in your own life. In all likelihood, you will find yourself beginning with the most *recent* events first. This is what we call *reverse chronology* and is the way most patients present their own histories. As clinicians, our task is to reorder the history into *true chronology*, which begins at the start of symptoms and proceeds to the present. This timeline approach to history taking almost invariably requires our skill in gently but firmly redirecting the patient's thought processes. At times it necessitates asking the patient to consider his illness in a far more general context (in terms of his entire life history) than he may be used to. Success depends largely on the skilled use of interviewing techniques, some of which work more effectively than others. The objective is to phrase questions in a way that firmly nudges the patient toward reporting symptoms in true chronology yet still maintains open-endedness and avoids putting words in the patient's mouth. Effective elicitors often include such questions as:

"Whén would you say you were last well?"

"Is thát the very first time you had that problem?"

"What happened thén?"

"What happened néxt?"

"What was the néxt major problem that happened after that?"

(Accents show words emphasized in speech)

These types of interviewer responses move the patient along *toward the present*. These imply linearity, progression, and timeline thinking. By contrast, there are times when the clinician wishes to elaborate a point before progressing. This can be facilitated by such interviewer statements as:

"Tell me more about that."

"Mm-hmm."

"Did you have other symptoms at that time?"

These questions tend to hold the patient at a stationary point for the purpose of expanding on details. A skillful interviewer uses both types of facilitating responses—returning a patient to the beginning, guiding him through a linear exposition of the problem, and stopping to expand on points when this is indicated.

Here is a clinical vignette that illustrates how skilled interviewing can help a patient achieve greater linearity in reporting his history. As the reader shall see, the student has her difficulties with the patient. It might be tempting to blame this on a "difficult patient" were the preceptor not subsequently able to turn things around:

A student recently found herself very confused about the progression of arthritic symptoms in an elderly woman. In fact, she could not determine the true onset of the arthritis, nor what the present illness actually was.

S: I'm Jan Holmes, a 1st-year medical student. As our preceptor told you, I would like to interview you and ask you some things about your medical problems.
P: I don't know how an old lady like me can help you (throws head back and laughs, slapping knee), but let's give it a try!
S: What is the main problem that brought you to the hospital?
P: I fell.

The student now has two tasks: to define the circumstances that surrounded the fall and to ask herself, "All falls don't land people in the hospital; what is special about *this fall* in *this patient*?" This is the *"why this person, why now?"* question, emphasized earlier in the book.

Picking up the interview:

S: When did you fall?
P: Last Sunday.

(Student mentally computes the number of days that have passed since last Sunday but fails to find out how long the patient has been hospitalized.)

S: Why did you fall?
P: I don't know, that's what you folks are supposed to be figuring out!

(The patient has properly warned the student about asking for the diagnosis.)

S: I mean, what were you doing at the time you fell?
P: Walking down the hall.
S: Did you trip?
P: No, everything just went black.

(The patient bails the student out by expanding beyond the *limiting* simple question.)

S: What do you mean, "went black"?

(Good! The student has used the patient's own words in an open-ended way to facilitate a response.)

P: Well, I had just been to the bathroom. I have such problems with my bladder, you know, and I got up to go to the living room. My husband was with me, and everything went black.
S: How long were you unconscious?
P: They said, just a few minutes.
S: Did you hurt yourself?
P: I bumped my knee and my head.

The student is searching for direction. She has deduced that trauma from the fall itself is probably not the main reason for the patient's admission, but her lack of knowledge of pathophysiology prevents her from determining what caused this patient to black out—did the patient experience syncope due to a cardiac arrhythmia? Postmicturition syncope? A seizure? Orthostatic hypotension due to dehydration or medications? A stroke? This list is not exhaustive, but it serves as a starting point from which a diagnostician could begin to rank data in the history according to their relative importance and thus guide further appropriate inquiry. At this point, the student who is knowledgeable about the seven dimensions of illness described in Chapter 8 would also be able to define associated symptoms (aura, palpitations, incontinence, or dizziness, for example). As has been mentioned, getting a good history of associated symptoms requires a fair knowledge of pathophysiology. This student, therefore, is stuck on trying to get the chronology:

S: Do you fall often?

(Dangerous. The student's judgment of "often" may be worlds apart from the patient's.)

P: Lord, yes. I was just in the hospital for the same thing.

(We still don't know what the patient's affirmative response to the "often" question above means, but now the student is strongly tempted to pursue this diversion in the hopes of getting a chronological account and perhaps some information based on an episode that had some closure, a feature painfully missing from the present episode as far as the student is concerned.)

S: What did your doctors say caused your fall then?
P: Well, I fell three times before they put me in.

(Correcting the student's assumption that a single fall had led to the hospitalization.)

S: When did those three falls occur?

P: I've been falling for a long time and they say there's nothing that can be done for it. It's due to the blood circulation in my head.

(The patient is having her problems helping this student but finally comes out with the diagnosis after all, at least in lay terms.)

If I was more active, I'm sure this wouldn't be happening, but the arthritis in my left knee has been killing me!

S: How long have you had arthritis?

P: For years. Dr. Baker has me on some experimental drug and has to keep me in the hospital to watch me.

(Chronology is a major problem here, but notice that the patient has sensed the student's difficulty and is much more open in terms of offering information to help. While it helps increase the amount of usable data, it strikes a serious blow to organization.)

It could be argued that the student ought to organize the data at this point into problems and pursue each one. A preliminary problem list following this type of assessment would rank the major problems as follows:

1. Falls
2. Arthritis
3. Bladder trouble
4. Compliance problems

Theoretically, each of these could then be pursued separately to get neat packages of organized data. But not only does the patient have difficulties with chronology, she also blends and dovetails the histories of *different* problems together. This intertwining of subjective data is the next major phenomenon we will discuss in this section.

The Patient With Multiple Problems

Patients with complicated medical histories, especially those who are elderly, often find it impossible to tell their stories in terms of isolated problems, out of the context of their whole life's experience. The student who attempts to unravel these stories can admittedly have a difficult time of it. Two or three illnesses may have similar symptoms, or may cause symptoms in several organ systems at the same time. No amount of skillful history taking will sort out and undo the dense intermingling of symptoms, signs, and feelings that patients with complicated medical histories experience. As Weed points out, to attempt to artificially force the patient into "clarity" would be like trying to read a book by reading all the odd numbered pages first, then going back and reading all the even numbered pages!

At such times, with such patients, students are apt to feel overwhelmed. A useful principle is—stick to chronology. Even a complex history will tend to become more comprehensible, if the clinician concentrates first and foremost on chronology, and lets the symptoms unfold as they may. The clinician can then go back over the data as need be to sort and group them into problems. Here is what happened later in the same interview when the preceptor took over:

Preceptor: Mrs. Jones, if you had to look backwards at the last time you were *perfectly well and healthy*, when would you say that was?
Patient: I've *never* been healthy!
Pr: Were you a 'sickly' child?
P: Oh, no! I guess I had the usual illnesses.
Pr: What about your teenage years?
P: I was OK.
Pr: After high school, did you maintain your good health?
P: Yes.
Pr: For how long?

(An important question. Up to now the preceptor has carefully led the patient through specific time frames, but now he jumps to asking the patient to think in summary terms over an undetermined period.)

P: Let's see, after I had my last baby I had my gall bladder removed.
Pr: How old were you at that time?
P: 41.

(Patient is 75 years old at the time of this interview—34 years ago.)

Pr: What happened then?
P: I was OK until my appendix ruptured.
Pr: That must have been a difficult experience.
P: Oh, my yes! I was in the hospital for 3 weeks.
Pr: Did you have any problems due to your appendicitis that showed up later?
P: Once, I had a blocked bowel that had to be operated on.
Pr: When?
P: That was in 1950.

(Quick mental arithmetic shows that this was 4 years after the gall bladder surgery—30 years ago.)

The patient is now smoothly on a chronological course, and while her perception is that she has "never been healthy," we have reduced our current unfilled timeline to the past 30 years and determined that she at least made it to middle age without any chronic illnesses. It is now more possible to refocus on the two main problems that seem to make up the present illness:

Pr: Did you have arthritis as long ago as 1950?
P: No, it began about 8 years ago.

(The patient has now captured the time frame that eluded her earlier.)

Pr: How did it begin?
P: At first my knees, then my back, hips and hands.

Pr: Has there been any change in the past eight years in the way the arthritis affects you?
P: It just slowly gets worse and worse.
Pr: Are the same joints affected?
P: Yes.

At this point, the interviewer would logically pursue directive and open-ended questions to define the course of this chronic progressive illness further. Here, we skip ahead and pick up the interview again just after the completion of questions related to arthritis:

Pr: It must have been during the problem with arthritis that you began having these falls?

    (A different problem, but attached to the time reference the patient did well with.)

P: Well, that's only been a problem for the past year.
Pr: How many times have you had these falling spells?
P: Let's see . . . altogether four times.
Pr: Did they occur close together?
P: I had three in one week, and one last Sunday, as I told you.
Pr: That must have been frightening to you.
P: I thought I was going to die.
Pr: How did you handle your fear?

    (An appropriate empathic diversion, the chance for which would be lost if delayed.)

P: I kept after my doctor until he admitted me.
Pr: When was that scary week?
P: The week before Thanksgiving.

    (Approximately 5 weeks prior to the interview.)

In a reasonably short time, we have found an 8-year course of arthritis and a 5-week course of syncope. The goal of chronology has largely been accomplished. In addition, we have been able to separate the two problems in the history although, as mentioned above, multiple symptoms may need to be recounted together by the patient to preserve chronology.

Beginning the History with a Patient Profile

Most patients are unfamiliar with medical terms. Therefore we urge talking with patients in plain English. Beyond the problem of vocabulary, however, is the threatening nature of the medical history itself. Virtually all patients are afraid—afraid they have cancer, afraid that they'll need an operation, afraid that they'll die. Plunging too quickly into the heart of the medical history can often be very threatening. In many cases its result is a hesitant, resistant, non-communicative patient.

Such a patient will understandably retreat into a position of aloofness and distrust, closing up to the physician and surrounding himself with a protective moat of repression and denial. The following exchange is an example:

Interviewer: Can you tell me about your headaches?

(Good open-ended question.)

Patient: They are severe, and ache across the front of my head.
I: How often do they occur?

(Chronology; no particular implied meaning.)

P: Everyday, all day.
I: How long have they been present?
P: About 3 months.
I: Have you noticed any other symptoms or feelings?

(Associated symptoms.)

P: No . . . like what?
I: Such as weight loss.
P: Weight loss?!

(Patient recoils from physician with a visible expression of shock and dismay.)

The interviewer here is considering depression as a possible cause of these headaches and is seeking positive or negative data pertaining to vegetative symptoms of depression (anorexia, weight loss, insomnia). The patient, however, equates the interviewer's question with the possibility of cancer! In a fleeting moment, the irritating headaches have "become" a brain tumor, a thought not far from the patient's mind even before the interview.

While there are appropriate times for dealing with the patient's worst fears about his illness, it is our belief that this time should usually be somewhat into the body of the interview, after an element of rapport and trust have developed. The present illness can and should be developed early in the interview, when patient and clinician are still relative strangers; but it usually should not be focused on *first*. Most patients are really quite extraordinary in their capacity and willingness to allow a virtual stranger (so long as he is involved in their medical care) into their most personal and private thoughts. We suspect this stems from many factors, including a somewhat altered state of consciousness that occurs in extreme anxiety. Whatever the mechanism, this is a very sensitive time both for data gathering and therapeutic effect. We believe that the patient, as a *person*, must be known to the clinician, and usually a patient profile is an excellent way to start. This reduces the subsequent strain of content-directed medical questioning and can be accomplished without undue delay in most instances.

Because it certainly is a subject that is very familiar to them, most patients are comfortable beginning a first encounter with a physician by describing a "typical day" and giving the physician a biographical sketch; their main concerns with illness will, in fact, relate to *how* it affects their lives. Asking for biographical information also introduces the patient to the process of thinking chronologically, which becomes so important later when the medical history is developed. In addition, a patient's general style of verbal and non-verbal communication emerges very clearly during a biographical sketch, more so than in a prematurely content-focused history. Similarly, the physician will be showing the patient facets of *his* style—including his capacity for warmth and interest in the patient—which might not emerge so clearly during, say, a review of systems.

In summary, then, it is usually advisable to begin an interview with the social history/patient profile before launching into the present illness. This prepares the patient for the medical portion of the interview both emotionally and cognitively; it reduces the likelihood of subsequent problems in communication; and it helps to establish a common vocabulary, and does so under non-threatening conditions. The outcomes will usually be increased rapport, communicativeness, and trust. Finally, experienced clinicians find, with great regularity, that the crux of a patient's medical problem lies in his life experiences, psychological reality, and emotional state. Clinicians who equate pathophysiology alone with "getting to the heart of the matter" run the risk of getting pathophysiology alone back from the patient; they may end up knowing what disease a patient has but not why he got it, why he got it *now*, how to help him with it, and how to prevent it from happening again. It is only through the integration of pathophysiology with an understanding of the patient that this more humane and effective kind of diagnosis and treatment can occur.

The following example illustrates such integration, showing the transition from chief complaint, to patient profile, then back to chief complaint again.

Doctor: What is the major problem you are concerned about?
Patient: I've been having stomach trouble.
D: Can you tell me about it?
P: Everytime I eat, I get a pain right here (pointing to epigastric area).
D: This looks like something you are quite concerned about.
P: It is!
D: We should pursue this, but first I'd like to find out more about you . . . are you from Denver?
P: Yes.
D: Born and raised here?
P: No, I was born in Alabama and moved to Chicago when I was 10.
D: Why did you move?
P: My father wanted to move North and look for work in a big city.
D: How many were in your family?
P: Six. I had two brothers and one sister.
D: Did you go to school in Chicago?
P: Yes.
D: How far?
P: Eleventh grade.
D: What did you do after that?
P: Worked in a laundry.
D: For how long?

P: About 2 years . . . it was to help with money for the house. My father couldn't keep a steady job.

D: Why?

P: He drank an awful lot.

D: How did that affect the family?

P: Well, he had problems with the law, and us kids had to take care of ourselves a lot.

D: What about your mother?

P: She never said much, but I know it bothered her.

D: What did you do after the laundry?

P: I got married and had some kids.

D: How many?

P: Three, one died at birth.

D: I'm sorry to hear that . . . how did that affect you?

P: Nothing much.

D: What do you mean?

P: Well, I cried at first, but later tried not to let it bother me.

D: Would you say it doesn't bother you now?

P: Yes.

D: I'm glad you can share these feelings with me. Are there people in your life who you can share your feelings with?

P: Not really.

D: It can get kind of lonely, then.

P: (Nods)

D: Tell me about your marriage.

P: It only lasted 5 years. I went on welfare after we broke up.

D: How long ago was that?

P: Three years ago.

D: What has happened to you in that time?

P: I tried to work, but babysitters were too expensive.

D: I can understand that. Are you still on welfare?

P: Yes.

D: Can you describe the place you live?

P: It's an apartment with two bedrooms.

D: Just you and your two children?

P: Yes.

D: Can you tell me what your usual day is like?

P: I get up with the kids, make their breakfast and lunch, then get them off to school. I do housework and watch some TV. In the afternoon I do a wash and talk to some friends. The kids are home at 3:00 and we spend some time together. We eat at 5:00 and don't do much after that.

D: How many meals a day do you eat?

P: One or two.

D: Do you eat meat or fresh vegetables every day?

P: When we can.

D: I know how difficult it can be to feed a family.

P: We do the best we can.

D: Do you have any hobbies?

P: I like to sew.

D: How about close companions or friends?

P: I don't have time . . .
D: Do you sometimes wish things were different?
P: Yes, I hate being so poor.
D: You've been through quite a bit in your life haven't you?
P: Yes.
D: And now to have stomach problems, too!
P: Sometimes I think someone has it in for me!
D: What do you mean?
P: Oh, this stomach of mine, all I need is an ulcer!
D: Why do you think it's an ulcer?
P: This pain.
D: Tell me more about the pain. . . .

Through open-ended questions and clear indications of empathic under-standing, the doctor has guided the patient through a brief social history/patient profile. The social and economic factors impinging upon this person appear quite important. Also of great value is the rapport building nature of the physician's warm and interested responses. The transition away from and back to the present illness was smooth and logical.

This psychosocial approach is a critical key to good interviewing. Human beings get illnesses within the context of their lives. It is incumbent on us as physicians to grasp the whole individual and approach him from the outset in a spirit that communicates this broad interest in him as a person. To do less is quite simply inadequate, substandard medical care. It continues to be unfortunately true, however, that during the course of medical training, students will see how frequently these values are forgotten, denigrated, and ignored.

References

Breslow, L., and Somers, A. R.: The lifetime health monitoring program. *N. Engl. J. Med. 296:* 11, 1977.

Voytovich, A. E.: Evolution of a non-threatening audit system in a large teaching hospital. In *Applying the Problem Oriented System*, edited by H. K. Walker, J. W. Hurst, and M. F. Woody, Medcom Press, New York, 1973.

Weed, L. L.: *Medical Records, Medical Education and Patient Care*, Press of Case Western Reserve University, Cleveland, 1969.

chapter 10

THREE PATIENTS

This chapter consists of interviews with three patients, all of which occurred in one of the teaching units of the University of Colorado Health Sciences Center. We have deliberately chosen routine encounters, not special cases. These interchanges are typical of the kinds of interviews and these patients typical of the kinds that students encounter in a teaching hospital. Of course, in a real sense, each of these interviews is very special, for each involves a unique person, in the grasp of a very critical life event; but we could have picked from a dozen others—they, too, would have been special. The uniqueness of each patient and of each doctor-patient interaction can excite, yet frustrate students. The diversity, variability, and unpredictability of patients attracts us to medicine; yet, it can be exasperating to realize that there are so few absolutes. "Classical" cases and "typical" interviews are useful abstractions, but they are more apt to be found on the blackboard than in the clinic. Students who hope to find the perfect interview in these examples will therefore be disappointed. Such an interview would be a fabrication.

Still, these interviews do make a number of interesting points that are true of almost all such encounters. First, experience does make a difference. The reader will quickly discern how much meaningful information can be obtained by an experienced and skilled clinician. Although very few interviewing tricks can be memorized cookbook style, there are abilities that can be developed. Second, in each of these interviews, the clinician and patient are from very different backgrounds, whether we define background as ethnic, socioeconomic, or professional (there is a vast difference between the special culture of a medical center and the culture of the rest of the world). Finally, in each of these interviews, the patient has a deep, yet understandably conflict-ridden wish to express something very personal to the physician. This wish is almost universal in patients. Physicians who come to appreciate the trust that this represents will feel rewarded by the intimacy and intensity that is so much a part of our work. Physicians who attempt to avoid the responsibility of this trust will find that it pursues them incessantly nonetheless.

We present the cases without comment, feeling that they raise more questions than they answer, and that this is as it should be.

Case 1

Bill M., a 28-Year-Old Man With "Hepatitis"

A group of four 1st year students is in its 5th week of an interviewing course. It is Tom's turn to interview, and he has been assigned Bill M., a patient on the general medical ward of a large V.A. hospital. Tom has been told nothing about Mr. M. (including his diagnosis) and has been instructed to concentrate on obtaining an account of the present illness and exploring the patient's concerns about his illness.

The group takes a few moments to locate Mr. M.'s room, which turns out to be one of the V.A.'s rare private rooms, located at the far end of a hall. A sign is posted prominently on the door that reads, "Hand Washing Precautions For Direct Contact." The preceptor, Dr. LaBedz, knocks at the half open door and then enters the room. After a brief exchange with the patient, he beckons the students to join them. They find a handsome, ruddy-complected young man lying on his side in bed. He has been reading a science fiction digest, which he now pushes aside. He smiles broadly and says, "Welcome! Come on in!" He appears to be in his late 20s and has a wiry physique, sandy-blond hair, and an angular, square-jawed face. His complexion is quite fair, but his face and neck are a dark, ruddy copper, suggesting someone who spends a lot of time outdoors. His blue eyes are alert, clearly tuned in to what is happening. In fact, he appears extremely well except for an i.v. slowly infusing into his left arm. In his room is a small color TV (probably brought from home), four get-well cards displayed cheerily on the windowsill, three thick paperback books (one of them is James Michener's *Centennial*), and three pots of flowers. In addition, there is a novelty card on his bedside table that reads, PLAN AHEAD

The students arrange themselves at the bedside in chairs, with Tom sitting directly across from the patient. Dr. LaBedz sits back slightly and positions himself so that he can observe both Tom and Mr. M. clearly.

Student: Hello.
Patient: Hello.
S: Can you tell me what brought you to the hospital?
P: My stomach.
S: Your stomach? Can you tell me about it?
P: Sure! Well, I started having pains in the lower part of my stomach, and the usual things didn't work, so I came to the ER.
S: When was that?
P: About 8 or 9 days ago.

S: How long had you been having this stomach problem?
P: You mean *this* time?
S: Yes.
P: It started with some cramps for a few days, then I couldn't have a bowel movement, so my wife and I tried some medicine, and it worked. Then I got nauseated and when it didn't go away, we thought it was another bowel obstruction, so we came to the ER.
S: How long did all of that take?
P: Before I came to the ER?
S: Yes.
P: About 5 days.
S: So the illness began about 14 days ago then?
P: Right.
S: What happened in the ER?
P: The doctor didn't know what was wrong, so they drew some blood tests, gave me Compazine, and sent me home.
S: Did you feel better then?
P: (Shifting restlessly now.) No, I got worse. We even tried to call the doctor for the blood tests results, but the doctor said they weren't ready yet.
S: When did you make that call?
P: (Sitting up now, with an angry expression.) About 5 days after I was in the ER, if you can believe that!
S: What did you do then?
P: I got so I couldn't hold anything down, so I came back to the hospital, and they put me in.
S: Did they admit you because of the nausea?
P: Yes, and the blood tests showed hepatitis.

During the following portion of the interview, the patient continues to smile and appears at ease with the group. In general, he seems healthy and happy, despite the fact that he is in a hospital with an i.v. running.

S: I'd like to go back to the pain for a minute. What part of your stomach was affected?
P: The lower part, on both sides.
S: What did it feel like?
P: Cramps. Kind of sharp.
S: Were the pains continuous?
P: Pretty much for a few days.
S: Did the pains move or radiate anywhere?
P: No, they just stayed down here (Pointing to lower abdomen).
S: Did anything make the pains worse?
P: Yes, when I tried to have a bowel movement.
S: What would happen?
P: The pain got so sharp, I thought I would pass out. My wife was really worried.
S: Did you do anything that made the pain better?
P: No. The usual meds didn't work.
S: Were there certain foods that affected this pain?
P: No. I was really unable to eat because I felt so sick.
S: You mean nausea?
P: Yes.
S: Can you tell me more about it?
P: Well, the nausea has been there all the time.

S: Did anything make it change?

P: No. It just stayed until I came into the hospital, then they gave me some medicine which helped.

S: Can you describe your diet to me just before you came into the hospital?

P: (Laughs.) I was lucky if a few sips of tea would stay down.

S: Did you lose any weight?

P: About 25 pounds!

S: What's happened since you've been in the hospital?

P: Well, I started turning yellow, then I began feeling better; but the doctors said my blood tests showed I was getting worse. That was about 2 days ago. Since then they've kept me on i.v.'s, and I'm getting better. I should be going home in a few days. (Smiles and looks expectantly at the group.)

S: Well, thanks, I think that's all the questions I have. Does anyone else have any questions? (The other students are silent.)

Dr. LaBedz: Thank you, Mr. M. Would it be all right if we left now and put our heads together a bit, and then come back if we have more questions?

P: Sure.

The students all say "thank you" and the group leaves. They find an unused conference room, pull up chairs around a table, and wait expectantly for Dr. LaBedz to begin the conversation.

Dr. LaBedz: Well, so what do you all think?

Tom: Well, I really think he has hepatitis. The history of abdominal complaints. The jaundice.

Preceptor: Did he look jaundiced to any of you?

Carol: Maybe a little.

Henry: I couldn't tell. I tried to look for that after he said he'd turned yellow.

Preceptor: I couldn't tell either. The lighting in the room was poor. How could we be sure?

Tom: Have him stand next to the window and look at his sclera?

Preceptor: Right. Our main purpose here is to interview, but it might be worth taking a closer look at his sclera. What else about the interview?

Richard: He seemed like a nice guy.

Carol: How do you mean, Richard?

Richard: Well, he was friendly and all. He smiled. He was clearly glad to be interviewed and to cooperate in our educational needs. By comparison, a lot of the patients we've seen are more sick, irritable, hostile. This guy was really tuned in, with it.

Preceptor: Well, what about that?

Richard: What do you mean?

Preceptor: Well, he may just be feeling better. For sure. But don't you think it's a *little* odd that somebody would be in a hospital, with an i.v. running, and *not* appear in more distress?

Carol: Do you mean, like, is he using denial?

Preceptor: Well, maybe denial. But anyway maybe that something, some emotional undercurrent, has been left out of the interview. It seemed kind of bland to me, considering how sick he really has been.

Henry: Don't you think we have to be careful though, not to make too much out of every little thing? He could just be in a good mood and feeling better. It doesn't *have* to be abnormal, does it, to be friendly and cheerful? (The group laughs.)

Preceptor:	So, you think I'm being too analytical? (The group nods and laughs again.)
Tom:	On the other hand. Looking back on it. He did seem to have some anger about how he got treated in the ER. Perhaps I didn't focus in on that enough.
Preceptor:	Good point. Any other observations? Is there anything else that we need to know about the present illness? (The group is silent for a moment, thoughtful.)
Henry:	Well, I thought he said a couple of times that he'd had this problem before.
Preceptor:	Right. What did he say?
Richard:	That he'd had the problem before. And also, I think he said something about having "another bowel obstruction" before. Didn't he?
Preceptor:	Yes he did. Do the rest of you remember hearing that? (The group nods.) So we really don't know what he's got now, or why. If he does have hepatitis, and that probably ought to be developed more fully too, it's still a physiologic diagnosis. It could have many etiologies and we don't know which one applies. Certainly, we'd want to know more about this history of bowel obstructions. Any other thoughts? (The group is quiet.)
Preceptor:	So we could say there are three things. First, we want to take a quick look at his eyes to see if we can observe the jaundice ourselves. Second, we want to develop this past illness a bit more and see if it relates in any way to the present. And finally—though it sounds like you don't all agree with me on this one—I think he was kind of bland. I'd like to get to know just a little bit more about him. Well, should we go see him?

At this point the group returns to Mr. M.'s bedside.

Preceptor: Would you mind if I asked a few more queuestions?
Patient: No, go right ahead!
Pr: Have you ever had hepatitis or jaundice before?
P: No.
Pr: Were you around anyone with jaundice in the pas. few months?
P: No.
Pr: Did you receive any blood transfusions in the past few months?
P: No.
Pr: What about travel outside the country?
P: No.
Pr: Did you use drugs of any kind by mouth or by injection?
P: I smoke pot once in awhile.
Pr: How about heavy drinking?
P: I don't drink.
Pr: Has there been any change in your stool?
P: No.
Pr: If you don't mind, at this point I'd like to see if we can move closer to the window and take a look at your eyes to see if we can see the jaundice. Is that OK?
P: (Laughing) Sure. You're only the eighth doctor in the last 2 days to do that!

Doctor LaBedz helps the patient over to the window, assisting him in navigating the i.v. pole. After careful examination of Mr. M.'s sclera in the brighter light, most of them feel they can see scleral icteris, though Carol says she's "not sure." After this, Dr. LaBedz helps Mr. M. back into his bed.

Pr: I'd like to return for a moment to something you mentioned before. You said you had had some problems with bowel obstructions. Can you tell us about them?

P: (Sits up in bed now, definitely looking more anxious and pensive. He shifts in bed as if to prepare himself for a long story.) Where would you like me to begin?

Pr: (Smiling) A long story, huh? Why don't you begin at the beginning.

P: (Pauses, heaves a deep sigh, and then begins.) When I was 14 I had appendicitis. They operated on me. Everything went fine, but 8 years later I developed a bowel obstruction. They operated and said it was due to adhesions. (At this point Mr. M. stops, as if waiting for a nod or some other encouragement to continue.)

Pr: Hm, Hm. Go on.

P: I was OK for a few years after that until I had a self-inflicted gunshot wound to the abdomen.

Richard and Carol display an unmistakable expression of surprise. Henry and Tom are more poker-faced, but clearly the tone in the room changes and suddenly there is a nervous, awkward chill. Time seems to slow down to a crawl, and everyone, including the patient seems agonized yet paralyzed in the silence.

Pr: (Quietly) I see. That was hard for you to say.

P: Well, I'm used to it.

Pr: Still, I'm very impressed by your willingness to open up and share something so personal. Many people wouldn't be able to. Yet I sense that this must be very important in understanding you. (Sighs of relief around the room—the unspeakable has been spoken—but everyone is still on the edge of the chair.)

P: Well, I know you need to know it.

Pr: Tell us about it. What was happening in your life then?

P: Well, it all began when I caught my wife in bed with another man. We were farming some land in eastern Colorado . . .

The patient goes on to relate a story of progressive estrangement from his wife, divorce, battle over custody of their two children, and finally mounting depression that eventually led to psychiatric hospitalization. There he carefully planned out the suicide while behaving in a "normal way" that fooled everyone. He goes on to recall his thoughts at the moment he pulled the trigger. It was a 12-gauge shotgun, and he recalled a loud explosive retort, a feeling of being hurtled to the ground as though by a huge gust of wind. Yet, he was unaware of any pain. The patient is able to recount in great detail his thoughts as he lay on the ground. He was suddenly full of self-recrimination and grief-stricken at the thought of leaving his children without a father. Finally, he struggled across the lawn and crawled to a phone for help. The following 18 months were spent in the hospital, with multiple operations and vast medical complications from which he finally recovered. His life had changed greatly after this cataclysm. He drew closer to his parents for the first time in many years, remarried, and was in the process of resuming a farming career when he developed his present illness. The interview ends as follows:

Pr: You've said a lot!
P: I guess I did. I only hope this thing now doesn't turn out to be too serious.
Pr: You're worried about that, aren't you?
P: (Eyes visibly tear up.) I think I am. (More tears now.) I never cry—this is ridiculous. It's just . . . it's just . . . for so long things were so *lousy*. Now, at long last, I finally feel like I'm getting things together—my wife, the new job. And I can't help saying to myself, "My God, Bill, wouldn't it be just like you—everything's finally coming together, only for you to screw up and have it all turn bad again!" (Patient is now crying copiously. Preceptor and students sit in silence, allowing patient to cry, waiting for him to regain his composure.)
P: On the other hand, the docs tell me I will get better from this. I do see hope ahead. Yet you can't help worrying. You know—I'm so close to getting it together. I don't want anything to ruin it now.
Pr: I can understand. It sounds like you've fought a long battle, and a very successful one. I suspect it took a lot of courage. (Patient nods.) We are going to have to stop.
P: Thanks a lot, doc. It helps sometimes to talk.

CASE 2

Chest Pain in a Young Woman

The setting for this interview is Friday morning attending rounds. This is a fairly formal weekly conference in which the house staff presents an interesting or puzzling new admission to their attending. It is regarded as an important teaching function and is attended by medical students and fellows, as well as by house staff. Although the atmosphere is friendly, with coffee and donuts and lots of banter, the house officers take the conference seriously and prepare for it. Their attending, Dr. Reynolds, is a young internist on the faculty. He has the reputation of being reasonable and supportive but firm in his expectation of conciseness and organization. The intern, Dr. Bergman, therefore begins his presentation with a well-prepared oral case presentation, which he has outlined on 3 × 5 index cards.

Dr. Bergman: This is the first Denver General admission for this 24-year-old unemployed, single, black female admitted for chest pain to rule out a myocardial infarction. The chief complaint was chest pain and fainting, and the informant was the patient and the ER sheet. The patient was in her usual state of health until yesterday evening at 5 p.m. when she experienced severe, crushing precordial pain that lasted 20 minutes, did not radiate, and was associated with anxiety, sweating, and nausea. The patient was at a bus stop across the street from the hospital and began crying out for help. She had a transient syncopal attack as bystanders attempted to help her and she was brought to the ER. In the ER she was found to have a sinus bradycardia of 45 and intermittent chest pain. Because it was impossible to rule out an MI, she was admitted to the hospital. The patient has had occasional episodes of chest pain of a similar nature in the past, usually lasting a few seconds. She denies all other cardiac and respiratory symptoms. There is no history of syncope, but the patient has intermittent bitemporal aching headaches lasting hours to days and associated with nausea. These symptoms have occurred every few weeks for the past 7 years. She denies other neurologic symptoms. Past history fails to reveal any major medical illness, but the patient had a tonsillectomy at age 7 and a D & C 2 years prior to admission for dysfunctional uterine bleeding. She has had the usual childhood diseases, immunizations are up to date, and she denies allergies. She currently takes no medication. Family history reveals maternal diabetes and hypertension and asthma in one sibling. It is otherwise non-contributory. The patient does not smoke and is a social drinker. The review of systems reveals no significant information. On physical exam, the patient appeared anxious, tearful, and in moderate pain, holding her chest. She had an i.v. in her left hand. Her blood pressure was 120/80, right arm supine, pulse 64 and regular, respirations 16 and easy, and temperature 36^9. The skin was normal. The head, eyes, ears, nose, and throat revealed no abnormalities. The findings of note were benign: The neck showed no jugular venous distension, the carotids were full and equal without bruits, and the thyroid was not enlarged. The chest was clear to percussion and auscultation. Examination of the heart revealed a quiet precordium. The heart was not enlarged by percussion, and the apex beat was barely palpable in the 5th intercostal space in the midclavicular line. There were no heaves, lifts, or thrills. Auscultation revealed a regular rhythm with a normal S_1. S_2 was physiologically split and there were no murmurs, gallops, rubs, or extra sounds. The abdomen was flat, soft, and mildly tender in the subxyphoid region with no rebound or guarding. There were no masses or organomegaly. The remainder of the physical exam was negative including the neurologic, which showed no lateralizing or localizing signs. Laboratory showed a normal CBC, electrolytes, and urinalysis. Chest x-ray was normal. The electrocardiogram showed a sinus arrhythmia, but no other changes. It was our feeling that the patient had chest pain consistent with angina although her age makes this unlikely. Other possibilities included costochondritis and esophagitis. Our plan is to rule out an MI and proceed with evaluation of other non-cardiac causes of the problem. Her other problems include syncope, headaches, abdominal tenderness, history of dysfunctional uterine bleeding, and status posttonsillectomy, remote. She was admitted to the intensive care unit for observation for further syncope, which we felt was neither cardiac-related nor due to a seizure. The patient complained of no further pain after our initial evaluation and treatment with one dose of morphine sulfate, 6 mg. i.v.

Dr. Reynolds: That was an excellent presentation. (To the group) Any other thoughts?

Resident: I agree that she needed to be admitted. At the same time, her age does make an MI sound pretty remote. Is there a family

	history for heart disease? Is there anything in her personal history, such as rheumatic fever, that might have set her up for such an event? You did say that there was no diastolic or systolic murmur, didn't you?
Attending:	Dr. Bergman?
Dr. Bergman:	There was absolutely nothing to suggest a murmur on physical exam. No mitral snap, no bruits, nothing in the carotids. Nothing to suggest rheumatic heart disease on physical examination. And we questioned her fairly carefully about a history of rheumatic fever in childhood. It was negative, and I think she's reliable. About the family history, I agree with you. She does have a mother with a history of diabetes and hypertension; but, we went over this pretty carefully, and there was no family history for early MI's.
Attending:	(To the group) Any other thoughts?
Another intern:	I think it would be important to get a triglyceride and lipid profile on this woman.
Dr. Bergman:	They're in the works.
Attending:	Anyone else?
Medical Student:	(Sitting toward the back of the room, raising hand rather tentatively) What about hysteria?
Attending:	Well, I think that's an interesting thought. No one has mentioned the possibility that this whole picture could be explained on a functional basis. But can you tell us what you mean by hysteria?
Medical Student:	Well, somebody who has a reason to develop a physical symptom. Some sort of conflict or problem that could be solved by getting sick. We just don't know whether this is present or not . . .
Attending:	That's a very important point. We really don't know the answer, because at this point we don't know a great deal about this person, her lifestyle, her current situation. You're quite right.
Medical Student:	Well, anyway, you could consider that her fainting and pain were a hysterical reaction to something.
Dr. Bergman:	(With a hint of irritation) How do you explain her bradycardia?
Medical Student:	Ah, . . .
Attending:	It's true—the bradycardia hasn't been explained, and she did have a sinus arrythmia on her EKG. On the other hand, the bradycardia was apparently transient and has not recurred since she's been on the ward. Correct? (Dr. Bergman nods.)
Attending:	The sinus arrythmia—it's hard to know what that suggests, if anything. The point is—and you're all correct—you have to take something like this seriously. The admission was appropriate, I think we all agree on that. In general, it's a mistake to assume something is functional and forget about even bothering to work it up. On the other hand, I think the question of hysteria is important. We really don't know anything about this woman. Without that information, it's very hard to know from what perspective we should view this current problem. (Addressing intern) Did you get any personal history that would be relevant?

Dr. Bergman: Well, she's recently separated. Beyond that, we don't know a great deal since we've been trying to work up the chest pain, and she was only admitted last night.

Attending: I understand. What you might say, therefore, is that this should go on the problem list as a feature of the incomplete data base—something needing further pursuit. (Intern nods.) I would like to say something about this hysteria business. I have some personal objections to the term. First of all, even in a technical sense, you really should reserve use of the word in a situation like this to someone with a conversion reaction. I'm talking about glove and stocking anesthesias, sudden unexplainable paralyses, tunnel vision—that sort of thing. Psychiatrists do use the term to describe a more general personality type, but I think we ought to be cautious here. Doctors tend to use these words in a way that has a disparaging, judgmental effect. (Addressing medical student) I know you didn't intend it that way, but I think jargon of this kind can sometimes get us into an unproductive sort of name calling. I'd prefer, in this case, to raise the question of whether psychological factors may have contributed to the current picture we see. And I think there's good reason to suspect that, though we also have to work it up carefully from a medical point of view. Any other thoughts? (The group is silent.) Then, why don't we go see her?

At this point, Dr. Reynolds and the group of 12 go to the intensive care unit and surround the patient's bedside. The resident physician stands closest to Dr. Reynolds. The interns come next. At the furthest point from the attending, the medical students cluster in and try to get a view. Dr. Reynolds stands facing the patient at her left shoulder. She is lying on her back in bed with the sheets pulled up in a veil-like fashion over her nose. Her eyes are closed tightly enough to make her eyelids quiver. She does not acknowledge the group's presence, but is clearly not asleep.

Attending: (Sits in a chair at the bedside and leans towards the patient.) Hello, I'm Dr. Reynolds, the attending doctor working with Dr. Bergman and the other doctors taking care of you here in the hospital.

Patient: (Inaudible whisper)

A: This is quite a place to find yourself in. Were you able to get any sleep last night or did all the activity, exams, and monitors keep you awake?

P: (In a near whisper, without changing her position) A little.

A: I know it must be hard for you to look, but I'd like you to know that there's a group of about 12 doctors standing around your bed. You don't have to look, but I figured you'd want to know that.

P: Um-hmm.

A: Before we came in, Dr. Bergman told me about what happened to you yesterday, but I would like to hear from you directly, if I could, what the main problem was that caused you to come to the hospital.

P: I fainted. (Patient continues to hold sheet up, eyes are more tightly closed and quivering as she answers.)
A: Can you tell me more about that?
P: I was at the bus stop and just fainted.
A: How were you feeling just before you fainted?
P: I don't know.
A: Had you been feeling perfectly well earlier in the day?
P: Sort of. (Patient slides sheet down to reveal nostrils and peeks with one eye at the group for an instant.)
A: What do you mean, "sort of"?
P: Do I have to answer all these questions?
A: Not if you don't want to, but I have the feeling that you are very unhappy about being here, and I hope to be able to decide with the other doctors here how to best take care of you and get you home.
P: Um hmm. (Patient maintains stoic, rather rigid supine posture.)
A: I realize that this is frightening to you, being in this intensive care unit, and I'm sure it's embarrassing to have all these people around your bed staring at you.
P: (Silence)
A: Maybe I could find out some things about you.
P: (Long silence)
A: Are you from Denver?
P: Yes.
A: Born and raised here?
P: No . . . I'm from Oklahoma.
A: How far did you go in school?
P: To the 11th grade.
A: What did you do then?
P: I went to work.
A: What kind of work did you do?
P: I worked in a laundry.
A: How long ago was that?
P: Four years ago.
A: What has happened since then?
P: Well, I came here about 3 years ago . . .
A: Did you work here?
P: No.
A: How have you supported yourself?
P: The "state."
A: That's kind of tough, isn't it?
P: Yup.
A: Who else lives with you?
P: My two children.
A: How old are they?
P: Four and two.
A: Who is taking care of them while you are here in the hospital?
P: (Silence)
A: Are they with someone now?
P: I think so . . . I don't know.
A: Well, who was with them yesterday when you fainted?
P: My neighbor.

A: Are you concerned about them and where they are?
P: They're OK. (Patient is becoming increasingly tearful.)
A: I'm glad. Has your neighbor called you here?
P: No.
A: Can you tell me about what yesterday was like?
P: What do you mean?
A: Well. I'd like to know what happened in your life yesterday. What time did you get up?
P: About 9.
A: What did you do then?
P: Fixed breakfast and did a wash.
A: What then?
P: (Appearing annoyed) My "old man" and me sort of got into it.
A: What do you mean?
P: He came to try to take the kids . . . he said I wasn't a good mother!
A: How did that make you feel?
P: How do you think? Lousy!
A: What did you do?
P: Called the police . . .
A: What happened then?
P: He started saying I better not call them.
A: Did he hit you?
P: Yes.
A: With what?
P: His hand.
A: Where?
P: Here. (Slides sheet down and shows attending the side of her neck.)
A: That must have been a terrible experience. Has it happened before?
P: From time to time.
A: Where were the kids during this time?
P: Right there. They're kind of used to it.
A: What happened then?
P: The police came.
A: What did they do?
P: They told me they couldn't do nothin' because it's a family fight.
A: What happened next?
P: My husband left . . .
A: Then what happened?
P: Some social worker came . . . to talk about the kids . . . I never touched them . . . she kept asking all these questions . . . I thought she would take away the kids. (Begins to cry.)
A: (Gentle voice.) That was very upsetting.
P: (Crying softly)
A: When did you leave the kids with your neighbor?
P: A little later . . . I felt real sick. My neck felt like it would explode, and I got real sick to the stomach.
A: What did you do?
P: I came to the hospital.
A: To the emergency room?
P: Yeah . . . but I waited for 4 hours . . . I was hurting so bad that I couldn't wait any longer . . .

A: So what did you do?

P: Got up and went to take a bus to another hospital . . . and then I forget. I guess I fainted . . .

A: That's quite a day! I guess in a way you're lucky you're here.

P: Yup.

A: At this point, with your permission, I'd like to examine you briefly. Is that all right? (Patient nods.)

At this point, the attending performs a brief examination of the patient's heart and lungs, taking special care to preserve her privacy by covering her breasts with a sheet. Finally, with the patient supine, he informs her that he is going to lower the sheet for a moment to feel for tenderness on her chest. He carefully presses with the tips of his fingers against her breastbone, just where the ribs connect to them. As he does so, the patient winces and gasps in unmistakable pain.

Attending:	I'm sorry I had to hurt you for a moment there. (To the group) Her cardiac exam is normal. But did you all observe the exquisite tenderness she displayed when I palpated her sterum along the costal sternal borders? How many of you have heard of Tietze's disease? (Most of the group nods.)
Medical Student:	Is that the same as costocondritis?
A:	Yes. What I do want you to know, since her findings are very suggestive for this, is that this is a syndrome that affects young people, especially when they're under stress, and it can be extremely painful. Although it's quite benign, it can be very frightening.
Patient:	I've had pain where you touched me before, but never that bad.
A:	(To patient) The pain you get with this can be quite bad, and therefore very frightening, though the condition is not serious. As I said to the doctors, it tends to get worse when someone's under stress, and it does sound like you've been under a lot of stress lately. (Patient looks straight ahead stoically and does not respond.) We'll also continue doing tests to make sure that there isn't another more serious condition to cause your chest pain, but my hunch is that that part of things will turn out OK. Still, it does sound to me like your life is in terrible turmoil right now.
P:	(Tears slightly, but does not respond.)
A:	This is not an easy time to talk about that, especially with such a large group. Yet I do think it will be very important for you to be able to talk about the stresses you are experiencing in your life right now. Perhaps Dr. Bergman and you can talk more later, when there's less of a crowd. I think that will be very helpful in allowing us all to decide how we can best help you.
P:	(Nods, still looking reserved, but now comfortable making eye contact with the attending and the rest of the group.)

A: Thank you for your time. We're going to leave now and discuss further how we can be of most help to you.

P: (Nods.)

CASE 3

A 45-Year-Old Woman with Headaches

A 45-year-old Mexican-American woman responds when the name, Marie Flores is called out in a crowded clinic waiting area. She appears deferential as she is ushered into an uninviting, institutional green examination room by a smiling physician, identifiable only by his countenance, a medical chart in his hand, and his shirt and tie. The two have never met, although the patient has been to the clinic several times before and the physician has worked there for 3 years. Upon reaching the examination room doorway, Mrs. Flores seems perplexed by her doctor's outstretched hand and finally grasps it only because he persists in this attempt to reach out, evidently a foreign experience to her. As she sits by his formica desk in a small vinyl chair, she glances warily at a crumpled sheet, pushed to the bottom of the examination table from a previous patient. The examination table is wedged into the only corner of the room in which it will fit. Still, the doctor evinces an unharried air, and his expression seems to connote genuine interest in her. The interview thus begins with a certain sense of surprise and hopeful expectancy.

Doctor: Hello, Mrs. Flores, I'm Doctor Paultz. I'm sorry you had to wait so long today.

Patient: Oh, that's OK

D: Can you tell me what the main problem is that made you come to the clinic?

P: Headaches.

D: Can you tell me about them?

P: Well, they just hurt ... I mean I don't know what's causing them ... and I feel kind of silly coming to a doctor ...

D: You feel silly?

P: Well, I usually only go to the doctors for colds and things, and ... well, I'm never sick!

D: It must be difficult for you to be here then.

P: Yes.

D: These headaches must concern you.

P: Well, they don't go away.

D: Can you tell me what the pain feels like?

P: I get this hard pain in the back of my head.

D: Hard pain? Can you be more specific?

P: It feels like someone is putting a band around my head and tightening it at the back, right here.

D: Does the pain move anywhere?

P: Yes, into my neck and around the side into my ... over here, my temples.

D: When did this first start?

P: About 3 months ago.

D: How often do the headaches come?
P: At the start they happened about once a week, but lately it's everyday.
D: How long does one last once it starts?
P: Anywhere from 1 hour to all day.
D: Do the headaches ever last several days without relief?
P: Yes, it was there for a solid week about a week ago.
D: You mean day and night without relief?
P: Yes.
D: That must have been very upsetting.
P: (Tears well up in Mrs. Flores' eyes.)
D: I can see that this has been very upsetting to you. It's all right to cry (handing the patient a tissue). Have you been able to share your feelings with anyone else?
P: (Shakes head, "no.")
D: Well, I'm glad you can do it now. It's very important to express your feelings. It can help.
P: I'm just afraid of what this could be . . .
D: What are you thinking of?
P: Oh, I don't know. Different people say things . . .
D: Like what?
P: Oh, you know . . . Like it could be something bad . . .
D: Like . . . ?
P: Oh . . . like cancer, or something.
D: We shouldn't jump to any conclusions. Nothing you've said so far makes me think of cancer; if we can work together, I think we can find a cause for your problem. Let's get back to the pain for a moment. You said the pain was there for a whole week a short time ago?
P: Yes.
D: If you look back over the 3 months, would you say the pain is worse now than it was when it started, the same, or better?
P: Worse.
D: In what way?
P: It's there all the time now, just about.
D: Has the feeling of the pain itself changed during the 3 months?
P: No, it feels about the same when it comes.
D: What can you do to relieve it?
P: Sit in a hot bathtub.
D: What else?
P: Aspirin used to help, but it doesn't seem to touch it anymore.
D: Have you tried anything else?
P: Not really . . .
D: What makes it worse or brings it on?
P: Sometimes nothing. Sometimes when I get angry or worried.
D: What kinds of things make you feel like that?
P: I don't know.
D: But you know when you're feeling angry or worried?
P: Sure.
D: Have you been to any other doctors for these headaches?
P: Yes, they said it wasn't anything!
D: What do you mean?
P: I had to go to the emergency room last week, and they said it was my nerves.
D: What did you think about that?

P: Well, I didn't think nerves could make a person hurt so much.
D: Did you say that to the emergency room doctor?
P: No, he was in too big of a hurry!
D: Did they do any tests on you?
P: Uh ... I think they took an x-ray and a blood test.
D: Did you find out the results?
P: I guess they were O.K. They never said anything about them.
D: Do you have any other symptoms during the headaches?
P: I feel dizzy.
D: Describe the dizziness.
P: Kind of drunk in the head.
D: Does the room ever feel like it's spinning with your dizziness?
P: No, I had that a long time ago.
D: How long ago?
P: Oh, Just for a day ... they said it was due to a virus. It was 10 years ago.
D: Do you have any symptoms with the headaches besides dizziness?
P: No.
D: What about difficulty with vision?
P: I wear glasses.
D: I mean, does your vision change during the headaches?
P: Not really.
D: What about nausea?
P: No.
D: Fainting spells?
P: No.
D: Numbness in any part of your body?
P: No.
D: Fever?
P: No.
D: Has this problem affected your appetite?
P: (Laughs self-disparagingly.) I don't think so! (Looks down at plump midriff.) I wish it would!
D: You mean you haven't lost any weight?
P: Right!
D: What about sleeping ... have you had any difficulty sleeping?
P: You mean because of the pain?
D: Yes.
P: No. I can always *go* to sleep ... even with the headaches.
D: I got the notion that you were having some sort of sleep problem, the way you answered that.
P: Well, I can't sleep all night.
D: What do you mean?
P: Well, I wake up and have a lot of trouble getting back to sleep.
D: Why do you think that is?
P: I don't know.
D: Is it due to the headaches?
P: No.
D: Well, some people who can't sleep are afraid to go to sleep ... they are afraid they'll die. Do you ever have that feeling?
P: Sort of.
D: Do you have dreams while you sleep?
P: Sometimes. I think I have one sometimes. It seems like I remember it when I first wake up.

D: Can you share the dream with me?
P: Well, I can't remember it too well.
D: Do the best you can. I think it will be helpful.
P: There's this dream . . .
D: Does it recur?
P: Yes.
D: How many times have you had it?
P: About four or five times in the past 6 months.
D: Tell me about it if you can.
P: I see my grandmother, and some other people.
D: Is your grandmother dead or alive?
P: She's dead.
D: When did she die?
P: Two years ago.
D: What do you see in the dream?
P: Well, everyone is walking around a big table . . . that has a lot of food on it.
D: Can you see the look on the people's faces?
P: No, but my grandmother turns to me and points my way.
D: What is she trying to do?
P: She wants me to come to the table with her.
D: What happens then?
P: I don't want to go . . . I get very scared . . .
D: Does the dream end there?
P: Yes, I usually wake up . . .
D: And have trouble getting back to sleep?
P: Yes.
D: Do the dreams have anything to do with the headaches?
P: I don't know . . . I don't think so.
D: I really feel like I'm getting to know you better, and I have more of a feeling that we can find out what's causing these headaches, but I need to ask some more questions to get to know you a little better.
P: Go ahead!
D: Are you from Denver?
P: No, from Trinidad (Colorado).
D: Did you grow up there?
P: Yes, but we used to spend a lot of time in Cortez (Colorado), too.
D: Who is *we*?
P: My sisters, my mother, and I.
D: What about your father?
P: I didn't really know him. They say he died when I was very young.
D: Did your mother raise you?
P: Not really.
D: Who did?
P: My grandma and her husband.
D: Where were they from?
P: Cortez. But, they really came from old Mexico.
D: Do you remember much about the times with your grandmother?
P: Sort of.
D: What did your grandmother usually do when you kids were sick?
P: She'd usually take care of it herself.
D: In what way?
P: Home remedies.
D: Do you mean herbs and things like that?

P: Sometimes.
D: Do you remember much about that?
P: Well, I know that she used to believe in the spirits very strongly.
D: What did you think about that?
P: I was just a little kid.
D: But what do you think now about it?
P: Oh, people say you can get sick that way.
D: What way do you mean?
P: (Hesitantly) . . . Oh, with prayers and the like.
D: Do you believe that?
P: I guess it's possible.
D: Do you remember your grandmother going to a special healer for herbs and prayers?
P: Yes, she went to a *curandera* in Cortez.
D: Did you ever go?
P: No.
D: But you know that she went?
P: Yes.
D: For what?
P: Oh, to get herbs.
D: Anything else?
P: Well, my aunt had a problem.
D: What kind of a problem?
P: Oh, I can't really talk about it.
D: You know, I understand that most Anglo doctors only treat sickness the way they are taught . . . but I have had some experience with the kind of illness we are talking about here. I know about what your people call the "special knowledge" . . . about the white and black magic, about *brujas* (witches). Was your aunt *imbrujada* (bewitched)?
P: They said she was.
D: Do you know who the *bruja* or *brujo* was?
P: They used to talk about her sister-in-law.
D: What did they say?
P: They said she was a *bruja!*
D: How did they know?
P: They always saw her around the house, and one day my aunt said a plate of noodles turned into worms! And it was right after this lady (the *bruja*) had been near the house.
D: What else?
P: This lady, she would come over at night and pluck one of my uncle's hairs, but each time she did it, she would turn a little older . . . you could see it in her face.
D: Did your grandmother try to help your aunt with the *curandera?*
P: Yes. They said prayers over my uncle.
D: Did they help?
P: Well, for a while.
D: What do you mean?
P: My uncle used to get very sick. They never found out what was wrong with him. I guess it was his gallbladder or something. Then he started to drink . . . he never stayed at home.
D: Did he leave your aunt?
P: Yes.
D: Because of this lady?

P: She was really jealous of my aunt for taking her brother.
D: Do you know if he got better after he left your aunt?
P: I think so . . . I don't know where he is now.
D: What about the *bruja*? Where is she?
P: I don't know if she is even around anymore.
D: Your aunt must have suffered a lot.
P: Yes, and my mother.
D: In what way?
P: She always hated that lady!
D: Was she good friends with your aunt's husband?
P: Yes.
D: Did your mother ever get sick because of the *bruja*?
P: I don't know.
D: Where is your mother now?
P: She died when I was 8 years old.
D: Of what?
P: I don't know.
D: Is it possible the *bruja* was responsible?
P: I think so!
D: That must be quite frightening to you!
P: Well, my grandmother told me never to worry about that lady.
D: Were you able to follow her advice?
P: I think so.
D: What about the dream you have?
P: I'm not sure . . .
D: Is it connected to the *bruja*?
P: Maybe.
D: Has anyone told you, or have you thought it yourself . . . that maybe a *curandera* could help your headaches?
P: Yes . . . my sister said so, but I don't know . . . I'm not sure . . . and I don't know of any *curanderas*.
D: What if I told you that I know one who I work with, who can talk with people and find out if they are *imbrujada*?
P: That would be good.
D: I'm thinking that the dream, the headaches and your memories about the lady in Cortez may be related. Do you think that is possible?
P: It could be!
D: I will set up an appointment with the *curandera*, if that's OK with you . . . and perhaps we can find out about any connection between these different things. But I still need to do a complete physical, some lab work, and a more complete history before we come to a final conclusion. Today, I want to do a partial physical to answer some questions I have about your headaches.
P: OK.

The physician does a problem oriented physical exam that includes examination of the head, eyes, ears, nose, and throat as well as a check of vital signs and a neurologic examination. Following the examination (which was totally normal except for tenderness of the scalp muscles) the interchange continues.

D: There, that wasn't too bad, was it?
P: No!
D: Well, why don't we make another appointment for a week or so. We really

need to help you with your headaches. At the same time we'll have your evaluation by our *curandera*.

P: OK.

D: It's been nice working with you today. I'm confident we'll get to the bottom of this.

P: Me too.

D: Good bye.

P: Good bye, thanks.

D: You're welcome.

The physician's problem list, assessment and plan appeared in the medical record like this:

Problem #1—Occipital Headaches

Assessment: The location of the pain, rather constant time/intensity curve over several months, persistence over days without relief, response to sleep, and the significant psychogenic factors (see Problem #2) suggest that this is a muscle tension headache. There seems to be no evidence by history or physical for vascular headache, sinusitis or a space occupying lesion with increased intracranial pressure. She is probably too young for temporal anteritis and the location of the pain and lack of temporal tenderness rule against this.

Plan:

Diagnostic: Finish history and physical.
  Basic lab profile.
  Work-up problem #2.
Treatment: No further Rx at present. Consider unified Rx approach with problem #2 to watch therapeutic response. Will consider relaxation training and analgesis next visit.
Patient Education: Work-up explained to patient. Consideration of link between psyche and organic disease begun.

Problem #2—Sleep Disturbance/Ethnomedical Problem

Assessment: Regardless of the organic nature of the headaches, the patient's cultural beliefs need attention in the total approach to her problems. This is true regardless of the culture. Her belief system seems well founded in her early childhood experiences, but her attachment to this cultural belief system, and therefore its relevance to problem #1, remains to be demonstrated. In support is her sleep disturbance, which has many of the elements of an Indian "ghost illness," i.e., dreaming of deceased persons who beckon the subject to join them. There is often unresolved guilt at the source, and one wonders if grandmother-mother relationship caused ambivalence in our patient, and also whether the patient's fears re: the grandmother being *imbrujada* as a result of battles with the *bruja* caused the patient to reject the grandmother. This could explain unresolved guilt or fears that the patient became *imbrujada* after the grandmother's death. The Indian-Chicano mix here is consistent with the cultural explanation for illness in the Cortez, Colorado area, and any ethnomedical treatment would necessarily be directed at the cultural expectation most embraced by the patient. In any event, the cultural influence on this patient's headaches is strongly suggested and must be considered along with the organic aspects of her problems.

Plan:
    Diagnostic: Consultation with the clinic's curandera.
    Treatment: To be determined following consultation.
    Patient Education: This process explained to patient as part of the
    medical interview. I will attempt to facilitate her understanding on
    future visits.

Appendix

THE ORGAN SYSTEM REVIEW

ORGAN SYSTEM REVIEW (O.S.R.)

A. General Health (constitutional)
B. Integument (skin, hair, nails)
C. Hematopoietic
D. Eyes
E. Ears
F. Upper Respiratory Tract (nose, nasopharynx and paranasal sinuses)
G. Mouth
H. Breasts
I. Respiratory Tract
J. Cardiovascular Systems
K. Gastrointestinal
L. Nutrition
M. Urinary Tract
N. Genitals/Sexual
O. Menses/Obstetrical
P. Musculoskeletal
Q. Nervous System
R. Endocrine System
S. Allergies
T. Emotional/Behavioral

The O.S.R. obtains medical information to assess a patient's health in areas that are not covered in the History of Present Illness or Past History. It is an organized survey designed to help the patient recall other significant medical problems, both past and present.

Rather than trying to list every potential medical fact available under each organ system, we have provided screening questions here for surveying each component. If the answers are negative, it saves the time needed to complete a "laundry list" and allows one to move quickly to the next component. If the answers are positive for either *past or present* problems, obtain the details, including whether the patient sought medical help, from whom, what was said, what was done, and what was the outcome.

Survey Questions

General Health (Constitutional)

1. How is your general health? (Other than any present illness)
2. How does your present weight seem to you?
3. How is your general strength and energy?

Integument

1. Do you now have any problems with your skin, hair, or nails?
2. Skin exposure and protection
   a. Do you sunbathe?
   b. What do you use on your skin regularly? Creams, lotions, etc.

Hematopoietic

1. Have you ever been anemic or had other problems with your blood?
2. Have you ever had any lymph node diseases?
3. Have you ever had a blood transfusion?

Eyes

1. Do you now have any trouble with your eyes or your vision?
2. Do you wear glasses? Why?
   a. Last time your prescription was checked?

Ears.

1. Do you now have any trouble with ear infections or hearing?
2. Have you ever had your hearing checked?
3. Are you exposed to unusual amounts of noise at work or with hobbies?
4. Do you have or have you had dizziness?

Upper Respiratory Tract

1. Do you now have any problems with your nose, throat, or sinuses other than the common cold?
2. Do you have nose bleeds?
3. Have you had chronic or recurrent hoarseness?

Mouth

1. Have you had any dental problems?
2. How often do you visit your dentist?

3. Have you had any recurrent or chronic sores in your mouth or on your tongue?

Breasts

1. Do you have any lumps or unusual tenderness in your breasts?
2. Any changes in the size or contour of either breast? Any change in either nipple?
3. Do you know how to do a self-breast exam? Do you do it?

Respiratory Tract

1. Have you had or do you have any problems with your lungs?
2. Is shortness of breath a problem?
3. Do you smoke?
4. Do you cough?
5. Do you raise phlegm?
6. Any tightness or wheeze in your chest?
7. When was your last chest x-ray?

Cardiovascular System

1. Do you have or have you had any heart trouble?
2. Do you have any chest pain, fatigue, ankle swelling, palpitations, or fainting? (Dyspnea was asked about under "Respiratory.")
3. Have you ever had an EKG?
4. Have you ever been told you had a heart murmur?

Gastrointestinal

1. Do you have any indigestion?
2. Do you have trouble swallowing, abdominal pain, heartburn, food intolerances, vomiting, diarrhea, constipation, bloating or tarry stools or blood in your stool?

Nutrition

1. Do you eat a well-balanced diet?
2. How many meals and/or snacks a day?
3. Typical diet in a day (include approximate amounts).

Urinary Tract

1. Do you have any problems related to kidney or urinary tract function?
2. How much fluid do you drink per day. (Estimate in 8-ounce glasses.)
3. How frequently do you urinate per day.
4. Specifically, do you have or have you had any of these symptoms?
   a. Any discomfort when urinating—burning or pain?
   b. Any frequency, urgency, or incontinence?
   c. Do you awaken at night to urinate?

    d. Males: any decrease in size or force of the stream; any hesitancy; voiding time increased; any episode of being unable to void?
5. Any flank or midback pain with or without chills and fever?

Genitals/Sexual

Genital

1. Have you had or thought you might have a venereal disease?
2. Any sores or growths on genitals, lips, or anus? Any associated rash?
3. Males: any urethral discharge or painful swelling of testicles?
4. Females: when was your last pap smear and results?

Sexual

Are you satisified with your sexual activity? If not, what is the problem? Are there any other questions you would like to raise regarding sex? (Note: The sexual history is important and requires tact. You will not obtain a sexual history if you do not ask for one; but you must be prepared to deal with the patient's concerns when he brings them up. Human sexuality is an important part of medicine and many medical schools now offer courses on it; further explication here is beyond the scope of this book.)

Menses/Obstetrical

Menses

1. Do you have any menstrual irregularities?
2. If past menopause, when did menses cease?
    a. Any bleeding since?
    b. Any menopausal symptoms? Any medications for them?

Obstetrical

1. How many pregnancies have you had?
2. Have you had any abortions or "miscarriages?"
3. Any complications or problems during your pregnancies?
4. Any birth control used?
5. If menopausal, when did your menses stop?
    a. Any bleeding or discharge since?
    b. Any symptoms you consider due to menopause?
    c. Any medication for menopause?

Musculoskeletal

1. Do you have any symptoms in your joints, bones or muscles?
2. Do you have any arthritis or "rheumatism?"
3. Have you had any fractures, bad sprains, or dislocations?
4. Have you had any back problems?

Nervous System

General

1. Have you had periods of disorientation or confusion?
2. Have you had any episodes of loss of consciousness?
3. Have you ever had a seizure (epilepsy)?
4. Have you ever had any infections of your nervous system (meningitis, etc.)?

Sensory

1. Do you have headaches regularly?
2. Any areas of numbness, increased sensitivity or unusual sensations?
3. Any problems with feeling or touch?

Motor Function

1. Do you have any weakness or paralysis in any extremity or part of your face?
2. Do you have any double vision?
3. Have you had any speech problems?

Coordination

1. Has frequent falling or a lack of balance been a problem?
2. Have you felt clumsy or dropped things?
3. Have you felt dizzy?
4. Do you feel stiff and shaky?

Endocrine System

Do you have any glandular or hormone problems?
If yes, *specifically* ask the patient about:
1. Thyroid
    hypofunction symptoms
    hyperfunction symptoms
    swelling, lumps, or tenderness over thyroid gland
2. Parathyroid
    symptoms of hypocalcemia
    symptoms of hypercalcemia
3. Pancreas
    symptoms of diabetes
    symptoms of hypoglycemia
4. Adrenal
    symptoms of cortical hyper- or hypodysfunction
    symptoms of medullary hyper- or hypodysfunction

Allergies

1. Do you have any allergies such as an itchy skin rash, hives, asthma, angioedema, food allergy, or seasonal pollen reaction like "hayfever?"

Emotional/Behavioral

1. Do you have any emotional or mental problems?
2. Do you consider yourself nervous or depressed?
3. Do you feel under stress a lot of the time?
4. Have you ever sought psychotherapy, or wanted to?
5. Do you have any other concerns in this area that you'd care to discuss?

Reference

Morgan, W.L., and Engel, G.L.: *The Clinical Approach to the Patient*, W.B. Saunders Co., Philadelphia, 1969.

INDEX

Adaptation
in medical school, 31–33
to illness, 78–84
Affect, as guide to themes in interview, 107, 116–117
Aggravating factors, in present illness, 175–176
Ambivalence, in patients, 62–64
Assessment, during the interview, 195–196
Associated manifestations, in present illness, 176

Biographical data, (*see* Patient profile)
Bodily location, in present illness, 174–175
Body language, 117

Cadaver
as patient, 26
as symbol in medical education, 21–27
Case history, use of self as a, 45–46
Chief complaint, in medical history, 170
Chronology
as dimension of the present illness, 173–174
as problem in data gathering, 199–204
Communication, in doctor–patient relationship (*see* Process)
Confidentiality, 99–100
Countertransference (*see* also Transference)
clinicians' reactions to, 149–150
definition of concept, 146

Data base, in POMR, 185
Denial
as problem in data gathering, 169
in illness, 53–54, 56, 63–64
of death, 23, 69
Discontinuity of self, in illness, 72–74
Displacement, 115–116, 126
Doctor-patient relationship
empathy in, 46, 81
importance of doctor to patient, 114
therapeutic potency of, 83, 96
three phases of interaction in, 193–199
trust in, 209–210

Egocentrism, in illness, 75
Empathy
definition, 135–136
for patients' anxieties, 106–107
in doctor-patient relationship, 46, 81, 100–101
Experience of change
in illness, 66–67
in medical students, 27–31

Facilitation, 127–133
Family history, in medical history, 177
First interviews
concerns about interrupting, 103
concerns about invading privacy, 102–103
concerns about professional behavior, 90–104
fears about patient crying, 103–104
guidelines for conducting, 104–108
natural abilities of students, 89, 96, 109–110
regulating psychological closeness, 100–102
role of preceptor, 108
student self-consciousness, 88–90
technical concerns about, 96–110
Follow-up
as part of POMR, 187–188
suggestions for, 160–162

Guilt
in illness, 75
in medical students, 22, 41–42

Humor
expressed in process communications, 116
in medicine, 40–41
Hypochondriasis, in medical students, 64

Identification
as distinct from empathy, 135–136
with patients, 89
Identifying data, in medical history, 167–169
Illness
altered state of consciousness in, 194, 205
as development, 59–61, 106

237